HEALING JOINT PAIN NATURALLY

HEALING JOINT PAIN
NATURALLY

~

Safe and Effective Ways to
Treat Arthritis, Fibromyalgia,
and Other Joint Diseases

~

ELLEN HODGSON BROWN

BROADWAY BOOKS
NEW YORK

Broadway Books titles may be purchased for business or promotional use or for special sales. For information, please write to: Special Markets Department, Random House, Inc., 1540 Broadway, New York, NY 10036.

BROADWAY BOOKS and its logo, a letter B bisected on the diagonal, are trademarks of Broadway Books, a division of Random House, Inc.

Visit our website at www.broadwaybooks.com

Library of Congress Cataloging-in-Publication Data
Brown, Ellen Hodgson.
Healing joint pain naturally: safe and effective ways to treat arthritis, fibromyalgia, and other joint diseases / Ellen Hodgson Brown.—1st ed.
p. cm.
Includes bibliographical references.
1. Joints—Diseases—Alternative treatment. 2. Arthritis—Alternative treatment. 3. Fibromyalgia—Alternative treatment. I. Title.

RC932 .B76 2001
616.7'206—dc21
                                                        00-049809

FIRST EDITION

Designed by Casey Hampton

ISBN 0-7679-0561-X

10 9 8 7 6 5 4 3 2 1

~ CONTENTS ~

PART 3: SUPPLEMENTATION THERAPIES

PART 4: REGULATION THERAPIES

HEALING JOINT PAIN NATURALLY

The Metaphor of Disease

Discomfort has meaning to the observing and reasoning individual. The intelligent man should see in all discomforts and pains hints or warnings that he should slow down and eliminate some of his indulgences.

—DR. HERBERT M. SHELTON,
Fasting Can Save Your Life[1]

Bodily afflictions, I have come to realize, can be blessings in disguise. They can prod us to greater heights of well-being and self-awareness.

First, in my case, there was menopause. Seven different gynecologists said I needed a hysterectomy—first for a prolapsed uterus, then for a large fibroid tumor, then for cysts on the ovaries—a dire recommendation that prompted me to research natural alternatives. I discovered plant-based progesterone and estrogen creams and other natural remedies, which not only reversed my symptoms without surgery but made me feel more mellow, more sensual, and generally more excited about my life than I thought I could feel in middle age. They also eliminated the carpal tunnel syndrome I had had for seventeen years, for which surgery had also been recommended. The crises of these threatened surgeries led me to natural correctives that took my well-being to new levels.

When my hip started to hurt, I wasn't too worried. I was confident that the body is the ultimate healer, and that if I could just figure out what it needed, it would repair itself. My pelvic bones had been fractured in a car accident at seventeen. After healing, my hip hadn't bothered me for the next thirty years; but by the time I was fifty-three it was keeping me awake nights. I couldn't seem to get comfortable in bed.

When I finally sought professional advice, X rays confirmed that I had a fairly advanced case of arthritis in the hip. The space between my hip bones on the right was significantly narrower than that on the left, which also wasn't as wide as it should have been. The doctor said he had seen many X rays just like mine, and that I was facing a hip replacement soon unless I did something radical to retard the process.

"I'm trying to scare you," he said.

"It's working," I conceded.

He suggested glucosamine sulfate (a popular nutritional supplement for building cartilage), stretching exercises, swimming or walking, a heel lift to correct an uneven leg length, and Aleve or some other nonsteroidal anti-inflammatory drug (NSAID) as needed for sleep. But I was already swimming and walking, and I was already taking glucosamine, which I had read about in the runaway bestseller *The Arthritis Cure.* And in my case, at least, it did not seem to be a cure—or not one of the noticeable, instant variety. As for anti-inflammatory drugs, I had done enough research to know they not only weren't cures but actually could make the condition worse by inhibiting the body's precious repair mechanisms. If I succumbed to NSAIDs for pain, I feared their repair-blocking action would indeed propel me into an early hip surgery.

I was opposed to drugs for another reason: I had become

convinced that disease is a message and a learning tool. If I dealt with it simply by suppressing the message, I would miss the lesson.

In the meantime, though, I needed some sleep. I heard about DMSO, a very popular remedy for joint problems—in horses. Although derived from wood, DMSO (dimethyl sulfoxide) was classified as a drug, and it was not FDA-approved for use in humans except for interstitial cystitis (inflammation of the bladder) and as a preservative in organ transplants. After reading the literature on it, however, I became convinced that it was a safer option than NSAIDs, so I tried it. I applied a rose-scented topical DMSO cream to my hip before bed and immediately slept through the night. Like conventional anti-inflammatory drugs, DMSO was only a temporary solution—I had to keep using it or the pain would come back—but it had the consummate advantage over NSAIDs that it did not work by inhibiting a natural function, and it had no demonstrated side effects.

But I still wanted to reverse the cause of my hip pain. I read that joint pain occurs at the sites of old injuries and other stresses because toxic substances accumulate in weakened areas (in my case the hip) and obstruct the capillaries, hindering the entrance of oxygen and food elements to the site. This produces inflammation, which produces pain by pressing on the nerves. I also read of successful reversals of the arthritic process through various detoxification programs designed to eliminate the accumulated toxins that are at the root of the problem.

Based on that research, I devised an eclectic home protocol that not only supplied the nutrients my body needed for repair (including glucosamine, MSM, pancreatic and digestive enzymes, and a range of other supplements) but aided the process by eliminating blockages to healing. Detoxification was done with fasting, homeopathic remedies, and a "niacin flush" that capitalized on the often overlooked eliminatory capacity of the skin. Meanwhile, I embarked on an exercise program that oxygenated the joints without overstressing them. To my delight, I was soon pain free and sleeping soundly without reliance on drugs of any form.

My hip gave me no more trouble for the better part of a year, until I danced the night away at several Latin parties in a row. (My family was then living in Guatemala, where my husband was posted in the foreign service.) My hip pain came back, but it wasn't just the hip that alarmed me. I had started to hurt all over. I had been in a car accident involving a whiplash the year before, and the headache and neckache from the "whip" had come back in force with an onslaught of new stressors. We were moving to a new post (Nicaragua); I was working on three books at once; and I had a toothache from a broken crown, but there was no time to see a dentist, as there was still the packing to do for our two-month trip to the States. Our daughter was to receive an award in Washington as a Presidential Scholar, an event that would have been the highlight of my child-rearing years if I hadn't suddenly ached in every part of my body. My hands were so swollen I could hardly use them, and I had absolutely no energy.

I had read that rheumatoid arthritis involves achiness and sore joints all over the body and that it can come on suddenly and be difficult to diagnose in its early stages. I feared I was developing that dire disease, until I came across a book by Paul Davidson, M.D., called *Are You Sure It's Arthritis?* Dr. Davidson stated that approximately a third of the diseases seen by rheumatologists and thought by their patients to be arthritis (inflammation of the joints) are actually soft-tissue rheumatic disorders (inflammation of the fibrous tissues surrounding the joints and sheathing the muscles). Predominant among these is one going by various names but now popularly called fibromyalgia. A technical diagnosis required three months of generalized achiness and joint pain, and mine had gone on for only two, but my symptoms were similar enough that I read on. Dr. Davidson said the condition typically comes on after a physical trauma that is locked in by stress. Unlike arthritis, which involves physical damage to the bones, fibromyalgia can often be reversed simply by rethinking the tension in the muscles and doing exercises to loosen them up. The pain comes from tension itself.[2]

Just reading those comforting words was enough to start my own healing process. My stresses weren't diminished, but my attitude toward them changed. I decided to relax into them, like riding a roller coaster with hands in the air. I would have faith in the maker of the machine and let the powers that be work out the details. I also went on a short fast and did some clay therapies (described in chapter 11), which broke the stress cycle by detoxing my body of built-up adrenaline residues. Remarkably, the problem went away. Besides a renewed respect for the power of stress to wreak havoc on the body, what I got from that unsettling experience was a sudden interest in researching both rheumatoid arthritis and the soft-tissue rheumatic diseases that mimic arthritis. The fruits of that research are presented in this book.

These two wake-up calls from my body prompted me to get serious about cleaning up my act. I became a natural remedies enthusiast, trying anything and everything I came across that was reputed to be good for the joints. Some of these remedies I won't discuss in detail because of their controversial nature. (One is hydrogen peroxide, which I actually thought helped. Another is live cell therapy, which is not FDA-approved in the United States but is available in Europe and in the developing world where I lived at the time.) The remedies available in the United States that I thought were effective are discussed in the following chapters.

The concept I finally developed through trial and occasional error was simple: clean the body from the inside out; eliminate blockages; stimulate energy pathways; nourish yourself. The body itself will do the rest. As a result of my adventure with arthritis, I now sleep free of hip pain, can do exercises I haven't done in years, and feel my strength and energy are recharged. My afflictions have again taken me to heights I would not otherwise have achieved. I'm so excited about these natural remedies that I want to share them in this book.

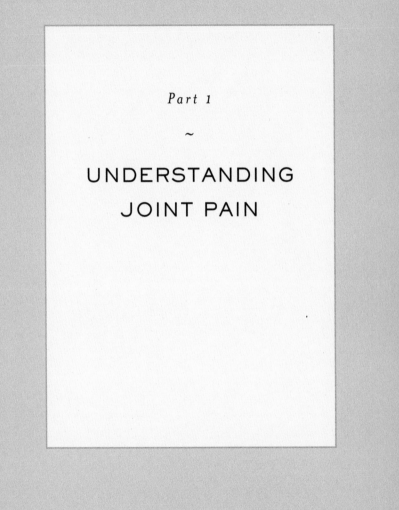

Part 1

~

UNDERSTANDING JOINT PAIN

ONE

Arthritis: The Disease, the Drugs, and Why Avoid Them

Physicians of the utmost fame
Were called at once; but when they came
They answered, as they took their fees,
"There is no cure for this disease."

—HILAIRE BELLOC (1870–1953)

Arthritis disables more people than any other chronic disorder and tops the list of diseases for which older people seek medical treatment. In 1998, the number of afflicted in the United States hit a staggering 43 million—15 percent of the population—up from 35 million in 1985, in part because the population in general is growing older. The market for analgesic painkillers is even more staggering, amounting to about $10 billion annually.[1]

Sales of Searle's arthritis drug Celebrex rivaled the blockbuster Viagra when it hit the market in early 1999. But the success of this "super aspirin" seems to reflect the widespread desperation of arthritis victims more than the viability of the treatment. Celebrex (discussed later in this chapter) is no more effective than older, cheaper options in reversing joint dysfunction. Its claim to fame is that it suppresses pain with fewer daunting side effects than the older drugs. Conventional medicine still has no safe and proven protocol for reversing arthritis.

DEFINING THE DISEASE

The word *arthritis* is derived from the Greek *arthron* for joint and *-itis* for inflammation. It thus means inflammation of the joint. Inflammation causes swelling, which causes pain by pressing on the nerves. Joint dysfunction that does not involve inflammation is technically called "arthrosis," meaning simply joint disease.

The most common form of arthritis is osteoarthritis, a chronic degenerative disease that is epidemic among the elderly. It afflicts about 21 million people in the United States. According to the Arthritis Foundation, the second leading arthritis-related condition is fibromyalgia, a form of muscular rheumatism that involves joint pain and is believed to afflict 3 to 6 million people. The third most frequent arthritic condition is rheumatoid arthritis, the most intractable and painful form of the disease. It afflicts 2.5 million people.[2] Fourth is gout, a gene-linked condition in which excess uric acid accumulates and forms crystals that irritate the joints. Other common forms of arthritis include bursitis, a painful inflammation of the bursae (the fluid-filled sacs that cushion the bones, tendons, and ligaments where they move against each other); and ankylosing spondylitis, an inflammation of the spine and hip joints. Many other conditions also involve an element of inflammatory arthritis, including systemic lupus erythematosus or SLE, a chronic inflammatory disease that strikes connective tissue throughout the body.

THE MECHANICS OF THE DISEASE

Different forms of arthritis have unique features that are discussed in later chapters. All, however, involve a breakdown of joint cartilage faster than the body can repair it. The joint is where the bones meet and are cushioned so they can move without irritating each other. The joint is protected by a capsule consisting of tough fibrous tissue. It covers the synovial membrane, which surrounds the joint and provides a lubricating fluid. Joints are covered with a smooth layer of cartilage that allows for easy sliding and absorbs shock. Arthritis strikes this cartilage, causing it to become swollen, flake, and crack.

When this occurs the body tries to protect itself by layering down extra calcium at the ends of the bone, forming bony spurs inside the joint. These are the bony knobs called Heberden's nodes visible at the ends of the fingers of some arthritis victims. If the node breaks off, it can form a "joint mouse" that moves in the joint space. A joint mouse that has gotten caught between the moving bones can cause serious pain. Friction between the bones also causes heat to build, but the narrowing of the synovial membrane makes blood flow insufficient to carry the heat away. When the joint isn't moving, the synovial membrane gets stiff, leading to "gelling" that makes it even more difficult to move.[3]

THE PHARMACEUTICAL APPROACH: NSAIDs

The conventional approach to the treatment of arthritis is to suppress joint pain with drugs. Aspirin and other nonsteroidal anti-inflammatory drugs (NSAIDs) relieve pain by blocking the inflammatory process, but this approach comes with a price. A 1998 study in the *Journal of the American Medical Association* estimated that more than 100,000 deaths now occur annually from legal drugs prescribed and used correctly. That makes pharmaceutical side effects the fourth leading cause of death in the United States, following only heart disease, cancer, and stroke.[4] And ulcers and gastrointestinal bleeding caused by NSAIDs are the most common serious adverse reactions of any drugs on the American market. This side effect has become so common and well known that the complex has its own name: "NSAID gastropathy." A recent Stanford study attributed 107,000 hospitalizations and 16,500 deaths yearly to NSAIDs. Taking them increases your likelihood of being hospitalized for gastrointestinal afflictions by a factor of more than six.[5]

People who take an occasional aspirin for a headache aren't at great risk. The problems come for people who take the drugs daily in relatively high doses over a period of years. Fourteen million arthritics now fall in that category. NSAIDs were developed specifically to treat rheumatoid arthritis, a crippling form of the disease for which side effect risks may be justified; but NSAIDs are now also frequently prescribed for osteoarthritis, a much larger market with a correspondingly greater potential for drug casualties.

ASPIRIN

Aspirin, the grandfather of anti-inflammatories, has long been the most popular treatment for arthritis. Americans collectively pop more than 80 million aspirin tablets daily. Critics question whether the Food and Drug Administration (FDA) would allow this drug on the over-the-counter market if it were introduced today because of its potentially serious side effects; but it has been around in pill form since 1899 (longer than the FDA itself) and was grandfathered in without testing.

How aspirin works wasn't discovered until more than seventy years after it appeared on the market. The mechanism involves natural substances called prostaglandins, which are released when cells are injured or stimulated. One type, called PGE2, alerts the body to disturbances in normal function by increasing the awareness of pain. Other prostaglandins contribute to the heat and swelling of inflammation and promote the coagulation of blood. Aspirin interferes with the body's biosynthesis of these prostaglandins, thereby suppressing inflammation and the awareness of pain.

The problem is that prostaglandins perform normal body functions that are suppressed along with the inflammatory process. Some prostaglandins help to regulate the flow of blood through the kidneys and the filtration and excretion of sodium and toxins. When aspirin inhibits these functions, the result can be fluid retention and the buildup of nitrogenous wastes in the blood.[6] Other prostaglandins have a direct action on stomach cells. They inhibit acid production and prevent acid damage to the lining of the stomach. When these prostaglandins are suppressed, acid can eat holes in the stomach and intestines. This unwanted side effect is the largest single cause of disease and death due to aspirin and other NSAIDs. Aspirin also causes an excretion of vitamin C in the urine that is three times normal; it can cause iron deficiency from blood loss from irritation of the intestinal lining; it prevents blood from clotting; and it blocks the effects of interferon, one of the substances by which the immune system fights off infections and other ills.[7]

NON-ASPIRIN NSAIDs

Non-aspirin NSAIDs include ibuprofen (Motrin, Advil), indomethacin (Indocin), naproxen (Naprosyn, Aleve), and piroxicam (Feldene), among other popular options. The non-aspirin NSAIDs were originally thought to have an advantage over aspirin in that they were better tolerated and produced less gastrointestinal distress. But the FDA eventually proclaimed that the safety of one NSAID could not be clearly distinguished from another.[8]

All NSAIDs, including aspirin, inhibit the synthesis of prostaglandins.[9] NSAIDs can also provoke asthma in some people. A British study found that people over sixty who took non-aspirin NSAIDs were three times as likely as nonusers to be hospitalized with bleeding gastric and duodenal ulcers.[10] In another study, elderly people who took ibuprofen regularly were found to be four times as likely to die from ulcers and gastrointestinal bleeding as those not taking it.[11]

Concerns about the side effects of NSAIDs have led the FDA to require new labels that state in part: "Serious gastrointestinal toxicity such as bleeding, ulceration, and perforation can occur at any time, with or without warning symptoms, in patients treated chronically with NSAID therapy." All of the currently available NSAIDs are now thought to have roughly equivalent pain-relieving effects, and all are known to cause stomach damage.[12]

Acetaminophen (Tylenol and other brands) is an over-the-counter analgesic that is easier on the stomach than NSAIDs; but it doesn't qualify as an anti-inflammatory, because it doesn't reduce inflammation. It therefore isn't much help for arthritics; and while it is easier on the stomach than NSAIDs, it still isn't safe taken over long periods, since it can cause fatal damage to the liver.[13]

ANTACIDS AND ACID-BLOCKERS

As many as 25 percent of people taking NSAIDs at any given time have evidence of ulcers detectable by clinical testing, but most of these ulcers have no symptoms and will heal on their own. The danger comes when an ulcer forms near a blood vessel or grows too large. It can then cause severe pain and other serious complications. Since in its early stages the ulcer goes unnoticed, a serious stomach bleed can come on suddenly, often requiring transfusions and surgery.[14]

Many arthritics try to avoid this result by taking antacids or acid-blockers (Tagamet, Zantac, Pepcid AC) preventatively. But a Stanford study reported in 1996 found that this could do more harm than good. The first symptom of an ulcer is usually heartburn. By masking heartburn symptoms, the drugs allow ulcers to get much larger before they are detected. People taking acid-blockers were found to be more than twice as likely to be hospitalized for gastrointestinal complications as those not taking them.[15] Acid-blockers also come with their own list of side effects, and one of them is joint and muscle pain. Again, they result largely because the drugs block natural processes.[16]

Stomach acid has beneficial functions, one of which is to kill bacteria in the stomach. Without the acid, you run the risk of infection by salmonella and other undesirables. Because acid-blockers don't cure ulcers but only mask symptoms, they have to be taken for life by ulcer patients. They have been called "annuity medicines" for drug companies, since they can cost several dollars a day.

COX-2 INHIBITORS

In an effort to circumvent the ulcer problem, drug manufacturers developed the Cox-2 inhibitors. These are "super aspirins" that block the Cox-2 enzyme that drives inflammation but don't block the Cox-1 enzyme that releases the prostaglandins protecting the stomach. The drugs don't suppress pain or reverse the ravages of the disease any better than older options, but they have fewer side effects than other arthritis drugs.[17]

At least, that is the claim of their manufacturers. The FDA is not convinced. It approved Searle's Cox-2 inhibitor Celebrex as a good option to relieve arthritis pain but declared there is no proof the drug is easier on patients' stomachs than other drugs. The FDA has required the same warning about side effects as for older painkillers.[18] Potential downsides of Celebrex reported in the *Proceedings of the National Academy of Sciences* include a reduction in beneficial prostaglandins and an increase in the risk of heart attack.[19]

Despite these drawbacks, in its first three weeks on the market in early 1999 about 142,000 prescriptions were written for Celebrex, making it the second-fastest-selling new drug after the anti-impotence drug Viagra. Over the long run, in fact, Celebrex is expected to fare better than Viagra, since most users take anti-impotence drugs only when the urge strikes them (or when they hope it will). Arthritis victims take arthritis drugs virtually every day; and once they start on one, they are likely to take it for life. In 1998, drug companies sold about $6 billion in brand-name prescription NSAIDs. Sales of Celebrex were projected to reach $1 billion a year later, equivalent to a sixth of the NSAID market.[20] Celebrex costs $2.50 to $3.00 per day for the lowest effective dose (200 mg). This is more than three times the cost of a therapeutically equivalent amount of NSAIDs (ibuprofen or naproxen); while glucosamine and chondroitin sulfates, the most popular nutritional remedies, may be had for as little as twenty cents a day.

Merck, the world's largest drug company, sought government approval for its own Cox-2 inhibitor, Vioxx, in the spring of 1999. Merck hoped to persuade the FDA that Vioxx is superior to Celebrex and does not need any warning label about gastrointestinal effects.[21] But as with Celebrex, the FDA has not permitted Merck to claim that Vioxx is less damaging to the gastrointestinal tract than traditional NSAIDs such as aspirin. The reviewing committee approved the drug for short-term use but observed that its side effects, including swelling, high blood pressure, and elevated potassium levels, increase with increasing doses, suggesting it might not be safe for use long term. The committee advised against its use for chronic pain and said its use for acute pain should be limited to five days, the longest Merck had studied it for that purpose.[22]

If the FDA is heeded, Vioxx won't be much help for arthritis sufferers, since they need long-term relief; but the FDA's warnings probably won't halt its use for arthritis pain. The rule is that once a drug has been approved, a doctor may prescribe it for any purpose deemed in his or her professional judgment to be appropriate. Celebrex, its competitor Cox-2 inhibitor, became the number one prescription arthritis medication a year after it got FDA approval.

THE UNDER-APPRECIATED BENEFITS OF INFLAMMATION

Even if the Cox-2 inhibitors are not hazardous to the stomach (a matter that remains in dispute), there is a more fundamental problem with these drugs. All arthritis drugs, including Cox-2 inhibitors, relieve the pain of arthritis merely by suppressing some stage of the inflammatory process, thus relieving pressure on the nerves. They do this by inhibiting the synthesis of prostaglandins that cause dilation of the blood vessels. The problem is that this dilation is necessary to increase the blood flow required for the repair of joint structures.

Studies have shown that suppressing inflammation not only doesn't cure arthritis but actually *speeds* joint deterioration. Inflammation is a natural process by which the body tries to remove dead or damaged tissue cells and lays down the matrix for new cells to replace the old. It does this by a buildup of body fluids that serves to destroy or wall off toxins and injured tissue and carry immune system cells to the site of damage. When this process is interfered with, the already compromised joint simply deteriorates more rapidly. In the hip, the resulting affliction is called "analgesic hip," a progressive degeneration of the joint caused by the very drugs given to treat joint pain. Cartilage and bone degeneration increases, leading to more hyperplasia (abnormal proliferation of normal cells), more joint capsule scarring, and more pain.[23] Animal studies have shown that aspirin, indomethacin, and other NSAIDs promote the rapid breakdown of cartilage.[24] All NSAIDs can also cause sodium and water retention, which is thought to trigger changes in deteriorating cartilage.[25] And NSAIDs suppress the production of proteoglycans, a type of glycoprotein found in connective tissue. The stiffness and cushioning ability of cartilage is directly correlated with its content of these substances.[26]

WHEN STRONGER MEDICINE IS NEEDED

When NSAIDs no longer work to suppress arthritic pain, corticosteroids (steroids) are prescribed. Steroids such as hydrocortisone, prednisone, and dexamethasone are powerful anti-inflammatories used by doctors to treat severe pain, but they can have correspondingly severe side effects. For rheumatoid arthritis, other strong drugs may be given, with even more serious side effects (see chapter 5).

When all else fails, the conventional approach is to replace the joint with an artificial one. That alternative, too, is fraught with risk. It is major surgery requiring a long post-operative recovery that can be painful and expensive, and that exposes the patient to serious hospital-generated infections. Surgery is an invasive procedure involving implantation of a foreign synthetic object into the body that does not come with a lifetime warranty. Artificial joints can last for years but not indefinitely; and by the time the patient is ready for another replacement, he or she may be too old to sustain the major surgery involved.

THE MARKET EDGE OF DRUGS

The bottom line is that conventional medicine has no cure for arthritis. It has a large and very lucrative pharmacopeia for suppressing symptoms, but these drugs can actually speed the destruction of the joints. Natural therapies are available that are safe and effective and that can actually reverse the course of the disease, as we'll see; but these remedies go untested and unheralded, because substances found naturally in plants or animals cannot be patented and are therefore not lucrative investments for manufacturers. Unless manufacturers can patent a product and recoup their investment, they cannot afford to put up the more than $100 million now required to get a single drug or device past the FDA. And until recently, manufacturers could not make therapeutic claims about products without FDA approval. New regulations have relaxed that standard, however, and natural remedies are now taking the market by storm. An array of natural products for arthritis is explored in Part Three.

While replacing drugs with nutritional supplements is a step in the right direction, this alone is not likely to reverse the disease. To understand what else is required, we have to first understand the cause. That question is examined next.

TWO

Osteoarthritis:
Finding the Cause

A disease known is half cured.

—THOMAS FULLER, M.D.,
Gnomologia (1732)

One reason arthritic damage has been considered inevitable and irreversible may be that most people with arthritis now take NSAIDs and other analgesic drugs for it, and these drugs have been shown to actually impede the body's ability to repair itself. Few studies have looked at the natural course of the disease without the use of analgesics and other drugs—few, but there are some. In one study, the researchers followed patients with advanced osteoarthritis who were given no drugs for a full ten years. Surprisingly, fourteen of thirty-one hips studied—or nearly half—showed remarkable clinical improvement and recovery of joint space as confirmed by X ray.[1] The difference between patients who recovered and those who did not involved something else besides drugs. Evidently, some lifestyle change was involved.

In the 1960s, Dr. Paavo Airola wrote in *There Is a Cure for Arthritis* that conventional medicine has failed to cure arthritis only because it hasn't yet recognized the disease's cause. Dr. Airola was a leading proponent of the naturopathic approach to healing. Naturopathic medicine is an alternative system involving a number of different modalities, including clinical nutrition, acupuncture, herbal medicine, homeopathy, and manual manipulation. What they have in common is that rather than suppress natural functions, they work to support the body's own efforts at cure. The first step in this endeavor is to understand what the body is trying to do.

TRACKING THE CAUSE OF OA

Osteoarthritis (OA) is conventionally attributed to the inevitable wear and tear that comes with age. When the cartilage cushion that keeps the ends of the bones from rubbing together deteriorates to the point where the bones grate against each other, inflammation of the joint occurs. Formation of the bony roughness known as osteoarthritis follows.

In "secondary" osteoarthritis, damage can be traced to an old injury, old fracture, tissue damage from disease, overuse of drugs injected into the joint, or occupational overuse. In overweight people, arthritis in the knees is traced to the extra burden their weight puts on those joints. Secondary arthritis can develop from a single traumatic injury experienced in youth, or from a less traumatic but sustained stress on a joint continued over a long period of time.

Far more common, however, is "primary" osteoarthritis, which just happens. You wake up one morning with it, with no identifiable precipitating cause. It usually hits suddenly, typically around age fifty; but X rays reveal that degeneration starts as early as age twenty.[2]

Under the wear-and-tear theory, the joints have just broken down over time. But this theory fails to explain those native groups following traditional lifestyles and diets among whom the disease is rare. Africans in the bush stress their joints daily, yet they generally manage to escape this "inevitable" wear and tear. Rheumatoid arthritis is also rare among these native populations. Heredity doesn't explain the discrepancies, since when these same Africans move from their villages to the cities, they are subject to arthritic disease like everybody else.[3]

Some scientists have blamed arthritis itself on heredity. They assert that about 6 million people with OA have a defective gene giving them a genetic predisposition to develop the disease.[4] But surveys have indicated that over 40 million Americans have arthritis, including 80 percent of people over fifty years of age.[5] If 80 percent of a population has a condition, it can hardly be due to an abnormal gene. The condition is normal. Looking for a responsible gene, like looking for a responsible germ, takes responsibility and control away from the patient and makes us victims dependent on doctors and drugs.

INEVITABLE WEAR AND TEAR
OR REVERSIBLE TOXICITY?

It used to be thought that cartilage could not repair itself sufficiently to reverse damage to the joints. Skin would regrow and bone would knit together again, but damaged cartilage just seemed inexorably to get worse. Clinical evidence that degenerative changes in the joints are not inevitable and irreversible came with the invention of the artificial hip. Research by Leon Sokoloff, M.D., involving hip joints replaced with metal implants showed that new cartilage could grow on the bone protected by the metal. Dr. Sokoloff concluded that the real problem is that stress on the joint keeps intervening and preventing this process. Cartilage can repair itself if given a chance.[6]

Evidence that OA is not the inevitable result of normal wear and tear on the joints was reported by a team led by Dr. Derek

A. Willoughby in England, who traced the damage not to raw joints rubbing together but to calcium deposits within the joints rubbing on and irritating them. An accumulation of unwanted calcium deposits is potentially reversible. When Dr. Willoughby's team examined the synovial fluid of 100 patients with osteoarthritis under an electron microscope, three-fourths of these patients were found to have tiny crystals in their fluid that turned out to be hydroxyapatite, the same mineral that makes bones and teeth. The effect was like throwing sand into the joint. The crystals irritated the rubbing bones, causing inflammation, tenderness, and swelling.

To make sure these crystals were in fact what was responsible for joint damage, the intrepid researchers proceeded to inject the crystals into themselves. Sure enough, the injected joints became sore and inflamed just as if the researchers had osteoarthritis; and inflammation increased with the amount and size of the crystals. The researchers concluded that the crystals, not the raw bones themselves, were what roughened the smooth cartilage, reduced its ability to cushion stress, and caused swelling.[7]

They hypothesized that these crystals were the result of an inherited disorder that impaired calcium balance in the blood. But again, the magnitude of the problem of joint dysfunction, which now strikes 80 percent of the American population over 50, hardly makes it sound like a genetic aberration.

AN ALTERNATIVE THEORY OF OSTEOARTHRITIS

Dr. Airola thought that OA is not a localized disease of particular joints but is a systemic condition that affects the whole body. Particular joints develop symptoms first only because they are the most susceptible to damage due to prior injuries or stresses. OA is caused not by normal wear and tear on the joints but by prolonged abuses involving faulty nutrition, overeating, a sedentary lifestyle, and emotional and physical stresses. The result is diminished vitality and resistance to disease, intestinal sluggishness, and an impaired ability to eliminate toxic buildup in the joints and soft tissues.[8]

Dr. Max Heindel, an early twentieth-century German writer, reduced aging to its most basic terms. He observed that the stages from youth to old age involve a gradual "ossification"—a hardening or calcification—of soft body tissues. This process results from the deposit of "ash"—earthy matter consisting mainly of phosphate of lime (bone matter), carbonate of lime (common chalk), and sulphate of lime (plaster of paris). The fact that arterial (incoming) blood contains more of this ash than venous (outgoing) blood indicates that ash is progressively deposited in the tissues, bones, and joints with the nutrients the blood carries. The source of this ash, said Dr. Heindel, can only be our food and drink. The result is a progressive increase in the degree of hardness and solidity in the bones, organs, and joints, which destroys the flexibility of the joints, muscles, and other moving parts; thickens the blood; and chokes up the tiny capillaries so that the circulation of fluids and the action of the system progressively diminish until death ensues.[9]

Later research confirms that extraskeletal calcification—the deposit of bits of calcium in normally soft tissues—characterizes most chronic disease. In coronary heart disease, bonelike matter is deposited in the vital arteries feeding the heart. In hypertension, calcium deposits clog the tiny capillaries in the extremities, preventing the free flow of blood. In the kidneys, they occur as kidney stones; and when the kidneys begin failing, they can appear throughout the arteries and internal organs. Atherosclerosis is the deposit of fat hardened with calcium in the arteries. In cancer, mineral deposits tend to be localized in the region of the tumor. In tuberculosis, calcium is deposited in the lungs. In the eyes, they produce cataracts. In bursitis, they occur in the bursae (sacs of fluid cushioning the joints). In scleroderma, calcified patches appear on the skin. And in arthritis, they occur in the joints.[10]

Research also confirms that the accumulation of extraskeletal calcium in soft tissues is related to lifestyle rather than heredity. In one study, researchers determined the degree of calcification in the aortas of seventy South African Bantus and fifty-eight Johannesburg whites who had died and had been autopsied. Calcium in the aortas of the Bantus had barely doubled between the ages of fifty and eighty, while in the whites it had increased sixfold—a difference of 300 percent. Whites over sixty-five years of age had three times as much calcium in their aortas as Bantus of equal age. Reflecting these differences in extraskeletal calcification, none of the Bantus had severe atherosclerosis, while ten of the whites did.[11] Again, these differences aren't genetic, since prosperous Africans frequently fall victim to coronary heart disease when they adopt American or European dietary habits and sedentary ways of life.[12]

Where does the calcium come from that settles in the joints and soft tissues? Evidently from the bones. Atherosclerotic calcium phosphate deposits have been found to have the same composition as bone. Their X ray diffraction patterns are indistinguishable from apatite, one of the two mineral constitutents of bones and teeth.[13] John McDougall, M.D., a professor at the University of Hawaii and the author of a number of popular books on nutrition, blames protein in the Western diet for weakening the bones by causing calcium loss. Protein is highly acidic, requiring calcium to buffer it. To do this buffering, calcium is pulled from the bones, not only weakening them but causing their joint surfaces to be more easily injured.[14] The calcium pulled from the bones to neutralize the highly acidic Western diet may also settle in the joints as extraskeletal calcium deposits, grating on the joint ends like sandpaper and roughening and damaging their surfaces.

On that theory, osteoporosis (age-related bone loss) is the flip side of the pathological buildup of calcium that clogs and hardens the joints and soft tissues in old age. Both result from our protein-laden diet, which leaches calcium from the bones. Americans have one of the highest calcium intakes in the world; yet our incidence of osteoporosis also remains among the world's highest, and so does the incidence of degenerative diseases such as atherosclerosis and arthritis involving the pathological buildup of calcium deposits. The good news is that this process seems to be reversible. The idea that degenerative disease is not inevitable and can be reversed reflects an exciting new paradigm in medicine, discussed next.

THREE

A New Medical Model: Seeing the Body as Self-Healing

The art of medicine consists of amusing the patient while nature cures the disease.

—VOLTAIRE

NSAIDs, cortisone, and other arthritis drugs are what Seattle researcher Dietrich Klinghardt, M.D., calls "suppression therapies." They suppress symptoms by chemically inhibiting the natural reactions and functions of the body. The assumption is that the body has run amok as a result of forces beyond its control—heredity or environment or invading bacteria—requiring science to step in and fix it. All conventional drug treatments—painkillers, antibiotics, chemotherapy, etc.—fall into the suppression category. They suppress the body's own functions and responses.[1]

There are, however, alternatives to this approach. Two other categories named by Dr. Klinghardt are supplementation therapies and regulation therapies. Supplementation therapies also involve popping pills, but in this case they are natural vitamins, minerals, or hormones. The assumption here is that the body is deficient in something, either because it is not properly making or assimilating that substance, or because of dietary deficiencies or blockages.

Regulation therapies, on the other hand, stimulate the body's own processes. Their goal is to unblock energy pathways and "stuck" functions so that the body can create its own hormones and otherwise respond as it was designed. Better-known practices in this category include acupuncture (using fine needles to stimulate the meridians or lines of energy running through the body) and homeopathy (involving "vibrational" remedies that re-tune the body energetically). Also in this category are Dr. Klinghardt's particular specialty, neural therapy (discussed in chapter 24); detoxification techniques that eliminate toxic buildup and remove blockages to the flow of blood and energy; and mind/body techniques that eliminate emotional blockages and address the consciousness element of disease.

While regulation and other body-supporting therapies are not actually new, they reflect an exciting new medical paradigm that is gaining ground mainly because the old one hasn't been working. Andrew Weil, M.D., a professor at the University of Arizona College of Medicine and a popular author and lecturer, attributes the current revolution in medical thinking to the health care crisis. The insurance system, he says, is breaking down. The situation has become desperate enough to prompt a willingness to look at alternatives.[2]

The prevailing medical model until now has been mere damage control—patching up holes in a leaking boat. This has been done by cutting out disease with surgery or poisoning it with toxic chemicals and radiation, in the hope that the disease would succumb before the patient did; or masking symptoms with drugs that turn off the pain constituting the body's alarm system, leaving the underlying fire to consume the patient. The drugs' side effects may even fan the flames, hastening his demise. The delight of the new paradigm is that rather than merely controlling damage, it can actually lead to greater heights of well-being. It sees the body as capable of healing it-self if given the proper building blocks and conditions. Disease becomes a metaphor, a signal to figure out what we're doing wrong, then do it right.

Cutting-edge medical doctors are now maintaining that de-generative disease is not only controllable but reversible. Deepak Chopra, M.D., another physician/author with a huge popular following, notes that in 1988, the notion that heart disease might be reversible was a revolutionary one. That was the year that Dean Ornish, M.D., a San Francisco cardiologist, proved that the fatty plaque deposits blocking the coronary arteries of advanced heart patients could be made to shrink using natural therapies alone. Before that, the official position was that heart disease progressed inexorably to the patient's death, no matter what he ate, did, or believed. The therapies used in Dr. Ornish's study were a strict low-cholesterol diet, meditation, and yoga. Since then, evidence has been accumu-lating that many chronic degenerative diseases previously blamed on irreversibly defective genes are actually diseases of civilization, which can be reversed by lifestyle changes, detoxi-fication, and the removal of blocks to strategic energy path-ways.[3]

UNBLOCKING AND BALANCING THE LIFE FORCE

While studies on the reversibility of chronic disease are new, the paradigm that relies on the body's own healing powers has been around for centuries. A flow of healing energy that allows the body to self-correct was recognized by Hippocrates, the fa-ther of modern Western medicine. His two most widely quoted maxims are "First do no harm," and "Honor the healing power of nature." Hippocrates called the healing energy *physis*.

Naturopathic doctors refer to *vis medicatrix naturae* (Latin for "the healing power of nature"). Chinese acupuncturists call the healing power *qi*. Indian yogis call it *prana*. Homeopathic doctors call it the "vital force."

Naturopathic medical systems see disease as a cleansing process, the attempt of a body out of balance to right itself. The appropriate treatment, from this perspective, is whatever it takes to put the system back into balance so the natural recuperative powers of the body can function unimpaired. How the therapist stimulates and balances the body's natural forces varies with the particular system being followed, but in all of them the underlying principle is the same. In acupuncture, it means stimulating the meridians, or lines of energy, that run through the affected areas. In chiropractic, it means adjusting vertebrae that may be affecting the nervous system and the body's natural defense mechanisms. In nutritional therapy, it means balancing the diet. In homeopathy, it means administering substances which, in healthy people in larger doses, produce the very symptoms of the patient; but in the patient in minute doses, stimulate the natural defenses and recuperative powers of the body.

The phenomena known as spontaneous remission and the placebo effect attest to the power of the body to heal itself under certain optimum conditions. But what are those conditions? Obvious factors include appropriate nutritional support, exercise, fresh air, sufficient sleep, and stress-free thinking. Toxic buildup also needs to be removed. Healing requires not only feeding and stimulating the life force but clearing a path so this force can get through. Naturopathic doctors maintain that the progressive hardening of soft tissues is reversible using various time-honored detoxification techniques. One is fasting, a period of time without food during which the body "cleans house." Another is inducing perspiration, which carries toxins out of the body through the skin.

The role of toxic accumulation from a bad diet is particularly evident in the form of arthritis known as gout, considered next.

FOUR

The Virtues of Temperance: A Look at Gout

May I govern my passions with absolute sway,
And grow wiser and better, as strength wears away,
Without gout or stone, by a gentle decay.

—WALTER POPE,
"The Old Man's Wish" (1685)

Dr. Herbert M. Shelton, another naturopathic doctor writing in the 1960s, reported seeing hundreds of cases of arthritis reversed simply by fasting—a period of abstention from food. He attributed all forms of arthritis to the same cause, which he called "toxemia"—the cumulative result of years of abuse "in eating, drinking, emoting, in sexual activity, and in other forms of activity." The result was an accumulation of toxins in the system. These toxins collected in the joints, damaging the cartilage and causing inflammation and pain.

"Rheumatism" is a term that covers a variety of aches and pains of the muscles and joints. "Rheumatism," like "rheumatoid arthritis," comes from "rheum," a mucus or catarrhal discharge like that from a cold or the flu. "Acute rheumatism" and "rheumatic fever" are acute aches and pains caused by an infectious organism. "Rheumatoid arthritis" is arthritis involving achy, flulike pains throughout the body. Arthritis is rheumatism involving the hard tissues (joints, bones, cartilage). "Soft-tissue rheumatism" includes conditions such as fibromyalgia and carpal tunnel syndrome (discussed in chapter 6).

Both arthritis and soft-tissue rheumatism result, according to Dr. Shelton, from irritation in the joints where metabolic wastes (the waste products of digestion) have collected. Pain and swelling follow. The body's immediate response to inflammation is an attempt to immobilize the area. The surrounding muscles and ligaments become stressed and contracted, producing an "on-guard" condition of tension that further increases the feeling of pain. When these pains develop in the joints, they are called arthritis. When they develop in the muscles, they are called rheumatism. Arthritis is more complicated and damaging than muscular rheumatism because it involves the cartilage that pads the ends of the bones meeting in the joint. Destruction of this cartilage can result in deformity. If the cause of irritation is not removed, the bones will finally join, or ankylose, becoming permanently immovable. Dr. Shelton found that the condition could be reversed with proper detoxification, however, if caught before permanent damage had resulted.

He concluded that the underlying problem in all cases of rheumatic and arthritic disease is an accumulation of toxic material at a faster rate than the body can metabolize it. Toxic material accumulates over the years in "enervated" people—people whose energy level is too low to dispose of the wastes of digestion. Enervation is caused by certain lifestyle habits, including overeating and eating the wrong types and mixtures of foods; indulgence in coffee, tea, liquor, and tobacco; draining emotional unrest; sensual indulgence; and lack of exercise. Dr. Shelton observed that arthritis sufferers are especially prone to overeating sweets and starches—breads, potatoes, cakes, pies, and candy.

THE LESSON OF GOUT

A clear illustration of the principle that joint pain results from an accumulation of waste products at a faster rate than the body can dispose of them is the form of arthritis known as gout. Gout (or gouty arthritis) is a painful arthritic condition caused by a faulty processing of uric acid, a toxic by-product of protein digestion. Although excess protein can precipitate an attack of gout, protein itself is not the culprit. Protein is a necessary component of the diet. Gout comes from *over*indulgence—eating more protein (especially red meat) than the body is able to metabolize at one time. Some people have a genetic tendency to reach this point sooner than most, but the problem is still one of balance and flow, of matching intake to the ability to metabolize.

Uric acid is usually excreted in the urine. In gout, it accumulates in the joint fluid and eventually crystallizes there, the way sugar crystallizes in water. These needle-like crystals settle in the joints and other tissues. When they settle in the kidneys, they can cause kidney stones; but their most common target area is the big toe (the end of the line gravitationally). The typical attack involves a sudden severe pain in a joint—the big toe, ankle, or knee—usually in the early morning. The joint swells and the skin over it turns purple. The pain tends to go away during the day and to come back at night, lasting for about a week. Repeated attacks can lead to destruction of bone. People may have gout without realizing it; the disease is often misdiagnosed as simple knee or foot pain. A classic sign that it is gout is that the feet hurt with the first steps in the morning.

Gout affects one percent of Americans, 95 percent of them men. While the tendency to develop gout is inherited, lifestyle is clearly a precipitating cause. Henry VIII had it. The disease is associated with affluence, meat-eating, and liquor-drinking.

Most victims are overweight. Gout can also be triggered by antihypertensive medicine and stress.

CONVENTIONAL TREATMENT

Drugs may be used to treat gout, but they can have unwanted side effects and don't address the underlying cause.

For long-term treatment, the drug most often prescribed is allopurinol. It stops the formation of stones and slows kidney damage by reducing the uric acid in the blood. Its drawbacks are that it can actually trigger acute attacks of gout when first used, and it can produce rash, hives, sleepiness, upset stomach, diarrhea, and headache.

The drug colchicine, a derivative of the meadow saffron plant, has been used for centuries by gout victims. It works by lowering the acidity of the joint tissues, thus increasing the solubility of uric acid and dissolving the uric acid crystals that cause pain. Because colchicine is very effective for gout but not very effective for other arthritic conditions, it may be used to establish a diagnosis in doubtful cases. If it works, the condition is presumed to be gout. Many gout sufferers swear by this herb-based alternative, but again, side effects have been reported from its use.

Aspirin, the conventional first treatment for other forms of arthritis, merely exacerbates gout, since it causes the *retention* of uric acid. But other NSAIDs don't have this effect and may be used. For acute attacks of gout that don't respond to milder drugs, corticosteroids may be prescribed; but again, users risk serious side effects (see chapter 5).

TREATING THE CAUSE

A safer approach to gout is to address the cause of uric acid crystal buildup. An obvious first step is dietary modification to reduce uric acid production. Many studies have shown the value of a diet free of meat, the major dietary source of uric acid, in relieving both gout and kidney stones. Uric acid and its salts are the end products of the breakdown of nucleoproteins, which come primarily from ingested animal products. Liver, kidney, brains, and sardines are particularly high in nucleoproteins. These foods are notorious for provoking acute attacks, particularly when overindulged in. Alcohol should also be avoided, since it inhibits the kidneys from eliminating uric acid from the body.[1]

As Dr. Shelton observed, however, the underlying problem isn't the types of food eaten but the quantity, resulting in a failure to metabolize them at a fast enough rate to clear metabolic wastes from the system. Not only do quantities need to be moderate but digestion needs to be adequate to metabolize food properly. Ways to improve the digestion, along with nutritional, herbal, and homeopathic remedies that can help gout sufferers, are discussed in Parts Two and Three.

The message of gout is to temper intake to suit the capacity of the digestive organs. Though heredity is a factor, control is still possible by regulating the lifestyle.

The message of rheumatoid arthritis is a bit more complicated. It is considered next.

FIVE

Beyond Wear and Tear: Rheumatoid Arthritis and the Autoimmune Factor

I am not suggesting that people consciously choose to have or not to have an autoimmune disease. However, sometimes illness is an indicator of an imbalance or dysfunction . . . [S]ometimes the first step on the road to healing is to understand one's disease as a metaphor.

— ALAN GABY, M.D.,
Townsend Letter for Doctors & Patients (1999)[1]

Osteoarthritis and gout are localized diseases, in which the rest of the body can feel good although the joint feels bad. Gout hits only the big toe, the ankle, the knee. OA, too, hits only one or two body parts first—knees, hips, fingers, neck, low back. It comes on gradually, begins only in a particular joint or joints or only on one side of the body, and does not kill (although the drugs taken to relieve it can).

Rheumatoid arthritis (RA) seems to be a different animal altogether. RA can come on suddenly and affects both sides at once. Although its most obvious symptoms are in the joints, RA involves the whole body, with symptoms ranging from fever, chills, loss of appetite, weight loss, and sweating to overall fatigue and stiffness. In its advanced form, RA is easily recognized, but diagnosis in the early stages can be difficult. The general feeling is one of the flu or of a chronic infection, but accompanying this whole-body achiness are sore, hot, swollen joints.

RA typically begins with pain in one of the small joints, usually the wrists or knuckles. Pain can then gravitate to the limbs, spine, and neck. Severe inflammation during an attack can erode the joints, causing irreversible damage. RA is marked by inflammatory changes in the synovial membranes and joint structures and wasting away of the bones. Carpal tunnel syndrome (tingling and pain in the fingers caused by compression on the nerves at the wrist) and Raynaud's phenomenon (unusual reduction in blood flow through the fingers on exposure to cold) are other common symptoms.

RA is a dangerous disease that in its most extreme manifestation can cause death or crippling injury. Fortunately, it rarely does. Twenty percent of victims recover completely, and for most of the rest, flareups are cyclical, interspersed with periods of wellness. Only 20 percent suffer permanent joint damage; and for all RA sufferers, the disease burns itself out and gets easier to bear over time. RA can strike at any age but favors the years between twenty-five and fifty. The fact that it affects women over the age of forty three times more often than men suggests a hormonal connection.

RA is an autoimmune disease, one of those baffling conditions in which the immune system loses its ability to distinguish between hostile and friendly fire and attacks the body itself. Inflammation of the synovial membrane lining causes the joint capsule to swell, thicken, and become hot. Cells rush to the joint to fight the inflammation, sometimes releasing an enzyme into the joint capsule intended to fight foreign invaders like bacteria and viruses. If enough of this enzyme is released, the cartilage and bones inside the joint can be digested and destroyed.

Besides RA itself (sometimes called "synovitis"), the term rheumatoid arthritis is used to describe several other diseases characterized by inflammation of the synovial membrane. They include juvenile RA, systemic lupus erythematosus (SLE), and psoriatic arthritis. Rheumatic fever, a related condition, is also an autoimmune disease. Other autoimmune diseases that can lead to arthritis include ankylosing spondylitis (an inflammation and stiffness in the spine and hip joints) and scleroderma (a connective tissue disease that causes the skin to harden and thicken). Fibromyalgia is a related connective tissue disease that also involves an overreaction of the body, a system apparently gone awry.

What causes the immune system to malfunction in these conditions? Research has focused on genetics. But while millions of dollars have gone into the pursuit of that theory, no cures for RA have resulted.[2] Again, the best that conventional medicine has been able to offer are drugs to suppress the symptoms of the disease. In this more serious form of arthritis, however, suppression generally requires stronger drugs with more serious side effects.

CORTISONE AND OTHER STEROIDS

One popular option is steroids, analogs of the hormones secreted by the adrenal cortex. Cortisone is an analog of a hormone produced naturally by the adrenal glands, which sit on the kidneys. When it was reproduced pharmaceutically and put on the market in the 1950s, it was considered a wonder drug, since it could bring immediate relief from pain caused by inflammation. The problem with supplying this hormone artificially appeared only later, as patients' adrenal glands began to atrophy. Those who took large amounts of it over a long period of time developed serious unanticipated side effects, including stomach ulcers, loss of muscle tone, "moon faces," a "buffalo hump" on the upper back, osteoporosis, diabetes, high blood pressure, nonhealing of wounds, cataracts, edema (swelling), increased appetite, depression, and psychosis. In addition, since steroids achieve their effects by suppressing the immune system, any infection is given a greater opportunity to spread.

The popular drug prednisone is a derivative of cortisone. A hormone of the steroid category, prednisone is a powerful suppressor of inflammation that has been used to treat a wide variety of rheumatic diseases. It is often used in low doses to tide a patient over until some other drug treatment kicks in. But this practice, too, can be dangerous, since oral prednisone is highly addictive; and its effects soon wear off, requiring use of a higher dose to get a response. At higher dosages, the result can be adrenal failure.[3]

For a single flareup, an injection of cortisone directly into a painful joint can produce dramatic pain relief without significant side effects. The inflammatory process is suppressed and the pain cycle is broken. But ice applications have been found to produce the same relief. And rheumatoid arthritis sufferers are dealing with more than the single flareup of a painful joint.

DMARDs: "DISEASE-MODIFYING" ANTIRHEUMATIC DRUGS

Some specialists believe that the progression of RA can be slowed if large doses of certain drugs called disease-modifying antirheumatic drugs are given early in the disease. These drugs include gold salts, given either by mouth or injection; hydroxychloroquine (Plaquenil), an antimalarial drug; penicillamine, a metal chelator; and chemotherapeutic drugs that suppress the immune response, such as cyclophosphamide (Cytoxan), methotrexate, and azathioprine (Imuran).

Use of the DMARDs for treating rheumatoid arthritis was discovered serendipitously, and their modes of action for the most part remain unknown. The *Harvard Medical Letter* has questioned claims that the traditional DMARDs reverse the disease.[4] Although people with RA tend to rely heavily on them, many patients experience little or no relief, and all of the drugs can have quite serious side effects.

Hydroxychloroquine or Plaquenil must be taken in high doses to be effective. These can cause irreversible damage to the eyes, resulting in blindness.

Immune-suppressing drugs cause damage to the bone marrow (resulting in blood disorders) and deterioration of the muscles.

Penicillamine is not an antibiotic, as the name suggests, but a drug made from the urine of people taking penicillin. It attaches to heavy metals and causes the body to excrete them. Apparently, it works on RA by clearing heavy metal accumulations from the joints (see chapter 26). It takes several months to begin working, when it does; and it can have disturbing side effects in the meantime, including explosive vomiting, gastrointestinal distress, sores, bone marrow problems, lupus, and myasthenia gravis (a chronic, progressive, and incurable neuromuscular disorder).

As for the gold salts, about 75 percent of users report feeling better after taking them. Grip strength is increased, morning stiffness is reduced, and X rays show that joint damage is actually slowed or even stopped. But levels of toxicity are so high that it almost seems to be a prerequisite for the success of the treatment. One-quarter to one-half of patients develop some side effects. The list includes skin rashes, blood disorders, kidney and liver damage, and (ironically) acute attacks of arthritis. The injections can also be painful and must be taken for weeks or months before benefits are apparent.[5]

Among newer options, a DMARD called leflunomide (Arava) was approved in 1998. Called a "pyrimidine synthesis inhibitor," it works by suppressing a natural process, arresting the growth of immune system cells called lymphocytes by inhibiting the activity of a certain enzyme. The drug has been shown to reduce signs and symptoms of RA and to retard joint space narrowing, structural damage, and erosions; but it can also have unwanted side effects, including liver problems, diarrhea, hair loss, rash, abdominal pain, back pain, and hypertension. Drugs called biological response modifiers have also been used on RA, but whether they produce long-term toxicity or alter the natural course of the disease remains unknown.[6]

NSAIDs: COMPOUNDING THE PROBLEM

Even the milder arthritis drugs—aspirin and other NSAIDs—can have more serious side effects for RA sufferers than for other users. People with RA have been found to have abnormally high intestinal "leakiness" or permeability. NSAIDs, which also increase gut leakiness, compound the problem. Increased gut permeability allows the absorption of molecules that should be too large to be absorbed. The immune system responds by binding these large molecules, called antigens, with antibodies. The resulting antigen/antibody complexes, called immune complexes, are then attacked and destroyed by compounds released by the immune system.

These immune complexes are called "the rheumatoid factor," a marker used to monitor RA. When they wind up in the joints and are attacked by the immune system, joint tissue gets destroyed along with them. The underlying problem may be food allergies, which cause the release of compounds that increase gut leakiness.[7] NSAIDs, which also increase gut leakiness, thus magnify a precipitating factor for RA.

THE FOOD ALLERGY THEORY

The food allergy theory is explained by Dr. Lauri Aesoph in *How to Eat Away Arthritis*. She observes that RA sufferers are frequently troubled not only with "leaky guts" but with low stomach acid. Low stomach acid and low digestive enzymes impair digestion, weakening mucous membranes and allowing unwanted toxins to pass through the defense of the gut wall and get into the bloodstream. Since poor digestion means that food is only partially broken down, the food particles passing through the gut barrier are unusually large. Consequently the immune system does not recognize them as food but thinks they are foreign invaders. System-wide immune reactions are then set off, in which immune system cells called lymphocytes are produced in great numbers and sent on the rampage. Excess lymphocytes wind up attacking weakened cells in normal body tissues. The joints are particularly susceptible, since they bear more stress than most body parts, and nutritional deficiencies cause them to be too weak to repair themselves at the rate they break down. Free radical damage to the tissues and joints also increases. Free radicals are highly reactive molecules with unpaired electrons that snatch up mates from nearby molecules. They are the sparks that fly from the oxidation, or burning, of food for energy. They are also used by the immune system to detonate invaders. Heightened immune system activity means heightened free radical activity.[8]

THE INFECTION THEORY

Food allergy is not the only theory of RA. There is also the infection theory, which attributes the tissue sensitivity resulting in symptoms to the toxins or protein products of invasive microorganisms or parasites. Infection is well known to cause other types of arthritis. Known infecting organisms include *shigella, salmonella, yersina,* and *chlamydia.* Reiter's syndrome is a type of arthritis in which the infection is still apparent at the time of diagnosis. It is usually treated with tetracycline antibiotics.[9]

The viral theory traces RA to a virus that penetrates into tissue cells. The immune system then confuses these cells with invaders.

RA has also been blamed on infection by parasites. A British physician, Roger Wyburn-Mason, found a particular parasitic amoeba in the tissues of all the RA patients he examined. He reported curing the disease by killing this parasite with drugs. But while Dr. Wyburn-Mason was a world-famous nerve surgeon for whom two different diseases were named, he was ahead of his time. When he announced that RA (a "known" incurable) could be cured, he was ostracized from the profession. Several doctors have developed successful protocols since, however, following Dr. Wyburn-Mason's lead. One is Gus Prosch, Jr., M.D., who reports a 75 to 80 percent cure rate with his patients since 1982. Another is Joseph Mercola, D.O., S.C., who reports a similar cure rate following a treatment developed by Thomas McPherson Brown, M.D., adding nutritional, antifungal, and food allergy components to the microorganism approach (see chapter 13). Also important to these protocols is overall body detoxification, including a dental overhaul to eliminate leaky root canals and mercury amalgam fillings, which are considered primary breeding grounds for infection[10] (see chapters 24 and 25).

THE DRUG THEORY

One problem with the microorganism theory is that no single microorganism has been found in all cases of RA. The theory also fails to explain *why* the immune system has gone awry and attacked normal cells along with infecting invaders. Homeopaths blame this phenomenon on antibiotics. They contend the drugs don't actually eliminate bacteria but just drive them deeper into the body, where they become incorporated into normal cells. These semiforeign cells are then attacked by the immune system, causing inflammation in the joints.

Alternatively, the foreign elements incorporated into the cells and attacked by the immune system may be the remains of bacteria killed by antibiotics but not disposed of because the inflammatory process has been suppressed by drugs. Drugs are much less efficient at disposing of invaders than the immune system itself, which eliminates them entirely. Detoxification of toxic substances is achieved naturally in the body by the coupling of two toxins, forming a new nonpoisonous compound that can then be excreted. This happens in the liver and connective tissues, resulting in acute inflammatory reactions. Detoxification may also be brought about naturally by coupling a toxin with a nonpoisonous substance, again producing a nonpoisonous compound that is excreted. Antibiotics kill bacteria but don't eliminate the remains, which stay in the body and can be absorbed into the cells.

NSAIDs make the situation worse by suppressing the inflammatory response, thus preventing the cleanup operation inflammation should effect. "Not-self" components are left behind, which are detected by the immune system and attacked as enemies of the body.[11]

Where the conventional theory sees the immune system as having "run amok" for unexplained reasons (generally attributed to faulty genes), the homeopathic theory maintains that the immune system is not at fault. It is simply doing what it is designed to do, rout out foreign invaders. Homeopathy is discussed further in chapter 27.

THE STRESS FACTOR

Another key causal factor in RA seems to be stress. Dr. Wyburn-Mason speculated that most people harbor microorganisms in their intestines and bowels that are capable of causing RA, but a healthy liver keeps the infection from doing harm. Infection spreads to the joints and blood only when the person's resistance becomes low and the functioning of the liver becomes impaired. Stress can inhibit the liver's ability to filter toxins from the body.

In mice, mental stress can actually kill by shutting down liver function. This was shown by Hans Selye, M.D., who discovered and mapped the "stress response" in the 1950s. Dr. Selye took two genetically similar mice and kept one in a small, cramped box long enough to make it visibly nervous and disturbed. The other mouse was allowed to run around normally. Dr. Selye then injected both mice with India ink. The unstressed mouse kept running around, exhibiting normal mouse behavior. The stressed mouse promptly died. The healthy mouse was then killed and both were autopsied. The healthy animal's liver was quite black, indicating it had effectively filtered out the India ink as it was supposed to do. The stressed mouse's liver was merely gray. It had failed to remove the India ink, which had asphyxiated the mouse.[12]

Research indicates that mental, emotional, or physical stress can also precipitate an attack of RA in humans. Stress causes the release of adrenaline and cortisone, a process that weakens the immune system. One study followed eight identical twins, one of each pair having RA. The twins without RA all reported they were not unduly stressed, while all but one of the twins with the disease reported that they were. Another interesting study found that psychotics never got RA. Only people who bottle up their emotions seem to be candidates.[13] Other studies are discussed in chapter 28.

SO WHAT CAUSES RA?

Underlying all of these factors in RA is a bad diet and poor digestion. These lead to a sieve-like "leaky" gut, which leads to food allergies, which lead to autoimmunity. Poorly digested foods wind up as too-large molecules that seep through the holes in the sieve. These oversize food particles are mistaken for foreign invaders by the immune system, which goes on the attack. Chemicals, pesticides, and other foreign residues on the food can also prompt an attack, and so can drugs and the germs and parasites that the leaky gut fails to keep from seeping into the bloodstream. Adrenaline released by stress further poisons the system. Joints weakened by nutritional deficiencies wind up being attacked along with the target toxins, since degenerating tissue is also considered foreign by the immune system. The whole problem goes back to the leaky gut, which goes back to poor digestion.

SIX

Arthritis Mimics: Fibromyalgia and Other Soft-Tissue Rheumatic Diseases

Every invalid is a physician.

—IRISH PROVERB

Although rheumatoid arthritis is the second most common form of arthritis, it has only one-tenth the incidence of osteoarthritis. A condition that is less well known than RA but is of wider magnitude is fibromyalgia. "Fibro" means connective tissue; "myo" means muscle; "algia" means pain. Fibromyalgia is a nonspecific pain syndrome of the muscles and connective tissue that cannot be explained by some other term like osteo- or rheumatoid arthritis. Fibromyalgia is an arthritis mimic that seems to be reaching epidemic proportions, affecting as many as 10 million people.[1]

Called by a number of other names, including fibrositis, myalgia, and tension rheumatism, fibromyalgia is a form of muscular rheumatism—an inflammation of the white fibrous tissue of the body, especially the muscle sheaths and fascial layers of the locomotor system. Fascia are thin sheets of connective tissue holding muscles, joints, and organs together. In fibromyalgia, inflammation is linked to the delicate balance between mind and body.

As already noted, the term rheumatism covers a variety of

disorders marked by inflammation, degeneration, or metabolic derangement of the connective tissue and joint structures of the body, characterized by pain, stiffness, or limitation of motion. Arthritis is rheumatism that involves only the hard tissues (bones, joints, cartilage). It can be imitated, however, by rheumatic diseases affecting the soft tissues (muscles, tendons, ligaments, joint capsules, bursae, and fascias). Soft-tissue rheumatic disease comes in many forms, including not only fibromyalgia but tendinitis, bursitis, and nerve entrapment syndromes such as carpal tunnel syndrome.

According to Paul Davidson, M.D., in *Are You Sure It's Arthritis?*, the amount of human suffering and disability soft-tissue rheumatism causes worldwide is truly staggering. There are an estimated 12 million sufferers in the United States alone. Yet this symptom complex has been called a "hidden disease" because it is hard to diagnose. Both hard-tissue and soft-tissue rheumatism can cause debilitating pain and stiffness, but soft-tissue rheumatism is generally easier to reverse, since it does not involve physical damage to the bones and joints. The trouble is that it is often mistaken for arthritis and is treated as if it were that disease, while the treatable underlying causes go unrecognized and unaddressed.[2]

FIBROMYALGIA

Tendinitis, bursitis, and carpal tunnel syndrome are localized types of soft-tissue rheumatism—the rheumatic pains you can "put your finger on." Fibromyalgia, by contrast, is a diffuse form of rheumatism involving both sides of the body. A mysterious autoimmune disorder having symptoms that resemble RA combined with chronic fatigue, fibromyalgia causes considerable pain and stiffness, yet laboratory tests routinely come out normal. It typically involves a physical stress of some sort compounded with emotional factors. Fibromyalgia may accompany arthritis and is more likely to strike where arthritis has already struck. In one study, 20 percent of patients seen at a rheumatology clinic had fibromyalgia, a category exceeded only by those patients with osteoarthritis (29 percent).[3]

Seven out of eight fibromyalgia sufferers are women, most commonly in their mid-thirties or at menopause. The main symptoms are persistent aches and pains, but the condition can also be marked by exhaustion, numbness, feelings of swelling in the joints, constipation or diarrhea, cold intolerance, disturbed sleep, tingling, and headaches. In addition, the syndrome usually involves emotional upsets—anxiety, tension, suppressed anger, depression.

Victims of fibromyalgia were once simply dismissed as neurotic. Today, even though the condition is recognized as a medical syndrome, the cause and cure remain mysteries. Fibromyalgia occurs when, for unknown reasons, the muscles start making too much fibrin—protein in the blood that the body forms into fibers, evidently to protect itself against traumatic injury. The fibrin is what makes the muscles painful to the touch.

Fibromyalgia usually begins when a person who is already under stress undergoes some further injury—the woman already run down with chronic fatigue or stress who gets in a car accident, has a bad fall, or contracts an infection. She thinks she is coping well, when suddenly she starts to have aches, pains, and stiffness throughout her body. At first it's only when she wakes up. Then it's all day, every day. She gets tingling in her arms, feelings of swellings in her hands. Her legs feel like lead, and she's exhausted. Fear that something degenerative and irreversible is happening makes matters worse. She goes to the doctor, but he finds nothing abnormal. Years ago he might have said it was all in her head. But today he is more likely to say that her pain is indeed in her body, not in her mind. Unlike arthritis, however, there is no physical damage to the bones and joints. Pain can occur without injury or tissue damage. Muscle tension alone can cause it.

To illustrate this possibility, Dr. Davidson described an exercise involving holding yourself with your knees bent, pressing your back against a wall. Soon your thighs will be in pain, yet no physical injury has occurred. The pain can be released by sitting on a chair and relaxing. The symptoms of fibromyalgia seem to be the result of an abnormal reaction in which the muscles respond to a combination of environmental and psychological stressors by remaining in a state of tension. The brain interprets this tension as pain, aching and stiffness. Says Dr. Davidson:

> If the stresses one experiences are so constant that the muscles have no time to rest, relax, and recuperate, the aches and pains themselves become a source of anxiety and stress, which sets in motion a vicious cycle of discomfort and misery. This is one "long strain" that we can prevent, often by interrupting the destructive cycle. The key is to provide our muscles time for rest and relaxation, allowing a period of repair and rejuvenation.[4]

The usual conventional treatment is merely symptomatic, involving analgesics, antidepressants, anesthetics, or corticosteroids that mask or suppress the problem without addressing the underlying cause. Recently, an alternative drug treatment has been developed for fibromyalgia involving glyceryl guaiacolate, the main ingredient in Robitussin cough syrup. Taken in very high doses over a long period of time, the drug dries up the fluids in the body and stops fibrin production. One problem is its side effects—including diarrhea, nausea, vomiting, and stomach pain—which can be more daunting than the disease.

Another problem is that for a large percentage of patients, it doesn't work. It is also an expensive and lengthy therapy that has to be used daily. If you skip a day or two, you're back where you started.[5]

A study published in *Arthritis Care Research* in 1999 found that almost all fibromyalgia patients are now turning to some form of alternative medicine, an indication that traditional drug treatment is inadequate for this baffling condition. The study suggested that these patients could benefit from acupuncture, homeopathy, manual-manipulative therapies, and mind-body therapies.[6]

Dr. Davidson's program for relieving fibromyalgia involves retraining—of both the muscles and the mind—to relax and release stress. It involves (1) education to understand the condition, (2) stretching exercises, and (3) appropriate relaxation. These techniques and other remedies for fibromyalgia are discussed later. He cautions that the diagnosis of fibromyalgia should not be made without a doctor's help, since it can be confused with some quite serious diseases requiring early medical attention.

LOCALIZED FORMS OF SOFT-TISSUE RHEUMATISM

Besides the diffuse form of rheumatism called fibromyalgia, there are the more localized forms including tendinitis, bursitis, and carpal tunnel syndrome.

Tendinitis comes from inflammation in or around a tendon, the band of tissue that connects muscle to bone. The condition usually comes from trauma and often goes away by itself after rest. Causes can range from a new pair of shoes that put unusual pressure on a tendon in the heel to an unusually intense activity involving the hands and wrists.

Tennis elbow involves pain in the elbow joint coming not

from the cartilage, as in arthritis, but from the tendons of the joint. Pain results when these tendons, usually accompanied by the muscles in the forearm, become injured or strained, most commonly from playing tennis.

Carpal tunnel syndrome or repetitive stress syndrome is pain, tingling, or numbness in the wrist, hands, and fingers, resulting when swollen or inflamed ligaments put pressure on adjacent nerves. Compression of the nerves of the wrist can in turn cause painful elbows or shoulders. Like fibromyalgia, this affliction is reported to have grown to nearly epidemic proportions worldwide, a phenomenon attributed largely to the explosion in computer use.[7]

The conventional treatment for carpal tunnel syndrome is to wear a wrist splint, especially at night. Pain relievers are also often prescribed. In the extreme case, surgery may be performed. None of these remedies, however, addresses the underlying cause. Even surgery may need to be repeated every few years. Vitamin B_6 supplements have relieved the condition in some patients, suggesting it can involve a deficiency of this vitamin.[8] Carpal tunnel syndrome can also be relieved by natural progesterone cream. These therapies and their implications are discussed in chapter 20.

Bursitis is inflammation of the bursa, a sac or saclike cavity filled with fluid that prevents friction between moving parts. Bursitis is most common in the shoulder capsule, big thumb, and hip bursae. Calcium deposits may contribute to the irritation. Bursitis or tendinitis of the knee can be confused with arthritis of that joint, while pain in the hip can be the result of a form of tendinitis called trochanteric bursitis that can accompany or be confused with pain from arthritis of the hip. The hip, like the shoulder, is a ball-and-socket joint. Muscles from the buttocks attach at the greater trochanter, the protuberance on the upper end of the femur constituting the ball in the joint.

Trochanteric bursitis results when the tendon attachments are inflamed. Typically the hip begins to hurt as you climb stairs or get up from a chair. You may be comfortable enough when sitting but find that after sitting for long periods, your joint locks up when you stand, keeping you from moving. At first, it will release after a minute, but this problem gradually worsens. The pain can also interrupt sleep.

While no one therapy works for every form of tendinitis, Dr. Davidson reports that some form of therapy or combination of therapies nearly always gives relief. Both rest and exercise are good—rest when the tissues are acutely inflamed and painful, exercise later to limber and strengthen them. Cold applications help in acute inflammation. Heat applications help relieve chronic pain by loosening the muscles and making exercise easier (see chapter 21). When exercising, tendinitis sufferers should avoid excessive strain. If stressful or repetitive activities are necessary, do them in short periods, resting in between; or condition yourself to the activity the way athletes do, pacing yourself and working into it gradually.[9]

SEVEN

Arthritis as Energy Blockage: The Perspective of Yoga

"You are old, Father William," the young man said,
"And your hair has become very white;
And yet you incessantly stand on your head—
Do you think, at your age, it is right?"

—LEWIS CARROLL,
Alice in Wonderland

Like naturopathic doctors, practitioners of the Indian science of yoga maintain that the various forms of arthritis are only different stages of the same basic affliction. Yoga is often thought of as merely an exercise routine, but in India it is an entire system of physical and spiritual health. Yoga means "union"—of mind and body, of mortal and God. In yoga science, the underlying affliction is described energetically, as a blockage of the flow of prana to the joints.

Prana is the circulation of energy in the body. If its flow is blocked or deficient over a long period of time, waste products of cellular metabolism and other toxic substances build up in the lubricating fluid of the joints rather than being efficiently carried to the skin and kidneys for elimination. Acidic wastes and toxins then irritate the sensitive nerve fibers of the joint, causing pain and stiffness, and the joint begins to deteriorate. The joint fluid dries up, the soft cartilage lining corrodes away, and the bones accumulate calcium that forms new bone and limits movement. Eventually, movement becomes impossible and the body becomes crippled and deformed.

In a book published in India titled *Yogic Management of Common Diseases,* Dr. S. Saraswati maintains that this process is reversible. If caught early enough, in fact, he maintains that arthritis can be completely reversed by yoga techniques; and even in severely crippled people who have already suffered seemingly irreversible damage to the joints, a daily regimen of yoga can effect remarkable improvements.[1]

VARIETIES OF PRANA BLOCKAGE TO THE JOINTS

Dr. Saraswati's summary of the varieties of joint pain and their underlying causes parallels naturopathic theory. Acute joint pain, he says, is a common symptom of many illnesses and infections, including colds, flu, fevers, and diarrhea. It occurs because viral or bacterial toxins released into the bloodstream accumulate in the joint fluids, blocking the flow of energy to the joints. Acute joint pain usually goes away as healing occurs. Rheumatoid arthritis is a rapidly crippling condition that often occurs in young to middle-aged people, involving a reaction of the immune system to an accumulation of foreign substances in the joint spaces. Gout occurs when the intake of proteins exceeds the body's capacity to metabolize them. Uric acid, a toxic by-product of protein digestion, accumulates in the joint fluid and crystallizes there. Osteoarthritis occurs in older people and results from a lack of regular exercise, sitting in chairs, overeating, and eating of rich foods (meat, animal fat, heavy fried foods, refined foods, synthetic foods, sugar, and salt), and constipation, causing sluggish elimination of the toxic end-products of this rich diet. OA often strikes first in joints that were injured earlier in life, the injury causing structural derangement and pranic insufficiency that were not completely corrected at the time. OA is also sometimes associated with an excess of extraskeletal calcium in the body, resulting from either a too-high dietary intake of calcium or an imbalance in its distribution due to parathyroid gland malfunction.

Besides lack of exercise and an overly rich diet, Dr. Saraswati says that mental factors may contribute to the development of arthritis. Psychic rigidity and tension—fear of letting go, inability to express emotion, and other subconscious tensions—cause a corresponding physical tension and endocrine imbalance. The result can be arthritis, rheumatism, fibromyalgia, and constipation.

Conventional medicine, says Dr. Saraswati, fails to address the underlying causes of arthritis. It merely treats the symptoms of pain and inflammation by suppressing them with drugs. Besides the hazard of side effects, the conventional approach blocks the useful biological functions that inflammation and pain were designed to serve. Pain tells us what is out of alignment and in need of rebalancing; and balance is the keynote of yoga.

YOGA SOLUTIONS

The natural approaches to cure recommended by Dr. Saraswati include:

1. *Asanas,* or postures, which put the joints and body through their full range of movement. The goal is to relax and massage them while avoiding strain and pain. Limbering up the limbs before attempting these postures by soaking them in cold or warm salty water is recommended to encourage blood circulation.

2. Breathing exercises, known as *pranayama.*

3. Techniques for relieving constipation, including specific

postures, dietary modification (reduce starches, increase fresh fruit, drink plenty of water), exercise after meals, cold baths.

4. A simplified diet, including: (a) cooked light grains and cereals (wholemeal bread, chappatis, rice, millet, barley, etc.); (b) boiled lentils (dal) for protein; (c) boiled or baked vegetables (especially green vegetables); (d) vegetable salads (leafy green vegetables, beets, carrots, cucumber, sprouted lentils and seeds, etc.); (e) fresh and dried fruits and small amounts of nuts; (f) avoidance of processed, synthetic and refined foods; reduction in intake of milk and dairy products; substitution of sugar with honey. If necessary, small amounts of white meats, chicken, and fish are allowed on this diet occasionally.

5. Spacing of meals to allow proper digestion between them. The recommended protocol is to eat only two meals a day, one between 10 A.M. and 12 noon, the second between 5 P.M. and 7 P.M. This ensures that food is in the stomach when digestive energies are high, and that digestion is well under way by the time you are asleep. Snacking or eating between meals should be avoided.

6. Missing a meal or fasting one day a week is recommended, especially to ease pain in acute conditions and accelerate relief and recovery.

7. Meditation to release pent-up mental and emotional tensions. One suggested meditation involves creating thoughts and mentally throwing them away, a procedure that aids in recognizing fixed and self-limiting attitudes and behavior patterns. Another meditation involves creating mental scenes where you express deep-seated anger and aggression while at the same time remaining a detached observer, thus releasing suppressed emotional conflicts that contribute to arthritic rigidity.

8. Appropriate exercise alternated with periods of rest. Rest is essential in acute arthritic flareups, but gentle exercise like walking, swimming, and gardening should be integrated into

the daily routine, along with yoga postures to maintain joint mobility and muscle strength.

9. Heat and massage. Hot baths and moist or dry heat applied to painful areas help relax muscles and loosen painful contractions. Heat also reduces pain and inflammation, increases metabolism, aids elimination of poisons, speeds the production of natural lubricants, reduces swelling, and aids in the reabsorption of undesirable calcium deposits and bone formations in and around stiff muscles, ligaments, and joints. Massage invigorates and relaxes the nerves and promotes circulation of blood and lymph.

10. A positive mental attitude. The yoga student is encouraged to try to be patient, think positively, and to think of his or her pains as temporary conditions that will soon pass with diligent yoga practice.

11. *Amaroli* (urine therapy). This practice is something Westerners have trouble with, but ancient Indian texts call it "the nectar of the gods." Gandhi attributed his health and longevity to drinking his first morning urine each day. For a Western treatise on the subject, see *Your Own Perfect Medicine* by Martha Christy, who used urine therapy to cure her own intractable case of lupus, an autoimmune disease of the arthritic type. Ms. Christy's book is thoroughly researched and cites hundreds of studies supporting the use of urea and urine therapy for healing. On the matter of sanitation, she explains that the kidney is a giant filter, and that urine is actually as free of infectious contaminants as distilled water. Urea, which comes from urine, is the basis of many popular pharmaceuticals, including Premarin (estrogen), one of the bestselling drugs on the market; and Urokinase, a high-priced heart drug.[2]

The Indian yoga prescription for arthritis treatment includes drinking one to three glasses of fresh urine daily, as well as massaging old or boiled urine into pain sites or keeping urine-soaked packs on them. The practice is said to be particularly useful in cases for which drug therapy has long been used and is no longer effective. Urine therapy is particularly recommended while fasting, to maintain strength and avoid hunger. The protocol is to omit a bit at each end of the urine stream and catch the rest, drinking all of the urine excreted until the evening of each day of the fast.

REVERSING TOXIC ACCUMULATION

The Indian system, like the naturopathic system, views arthritis as a disease of accumulated toxins in the joints, which can be reversed by techniques to eliminate those toxins and rebuild the joints. Nutritional supplements like the currently popular glucosamine are good and necessary for the rebuilding process; but to effect a real cure, cleanup techniques and dietary changes are also required. Fasting, a detox treatment older than the Bible, is the subject of chapter 8.

Part 2

~

ARTHRITIS, DIET, AND DETOXIFICATION

EIGHT

Fasting Away Toxic Buildup
in the Joints

*Fasting relieves the pains of arthritis . . . more effectively than
drugs and does it without risk of harm . . . Nothing can more
certainly or more rapidly alter the state of the nutrition of the
body than a fast. NO other means at our disposal brings about
a more rapid change in the chemistry of the body, especially of
its fluids and secretions.*

—DR. HERBERT M. SHELTON,
Fasting Can Save Your Life[1] (1964)

Fasting is not only one of the oldest but is still one of the best
ways to detoxify the body. Dr. M. O. Garten, a naturopathic
writer who was an avid proponent of this technique, said that
each time he tried it, "I always felt like shouting to the entire
world about this true panacea of recreating or maintaining the
genuine pleasures of living."[2]

Fasting is a period without food during which the body
"cleans house" and metabolizes waste products. The physical
benefits of fasting were discovered by Western naturopathic
medicine in 1880, when an eminent physician named Dr.
Tanner responded to a challenge to the Biblical account of
Jesus's fast. The challenger maintained that it was not possible to
survive a fast of forty days. Dr. Tanner countered that it was not

only possible but that the body would benefit from the feat. To prove it, he fasted forty days on water alone and came out feeling unusually well. He repeated this performance on two further occasions, and lived to be ninety-two. Shortly before his death he said that his vigorous health and long life, which had been free from the usual infirmities of age, were the result of his three forty-day fasts.

FASTING AND ARTHRITIS: THE EVIDENCE

Even if you do not want to try fasting to relieve joint pain, the research on it is illuminating. A number of studies now confirm that abstaining from food altogether for a period of time can relieve arthritis symptoms, indicating that something more must be involved than mere wear and tear on the joints.

Most of these studies involve rheumatoid arthritis. One was a Japanese study reported in 1999. Fourteen patients with RA undertook a three- to five-day fast three times during a fifty-five-day stay at the Koda hospital. When not fasting, they ate a 1,200-calorie vegan (no-animal-products) diet that basically consisted of unpolished rice gruel, juice of raw vegetables, soya bean curd, and sesame seeds. Objective measures of RA status in these patients significantly improved. The patients lost some weight, but their body protein levels stayed the same, indicating that the weight loss did not come at the expense of their muscles but of fat. The researchers concluded that fasting combined with a 1,200-calorie vegan diet can significantly improve the symptoms of RA without adversely affecting nutritional status.[3]

In a Swedish study, patients with RA who went on a total fast for a few days experienced a substantial reduction in joint pain, swelling, morning stiffness, and other arthritic symptoms. This remission subsided after discontinuation of fasting, but slowly.[4]

In a randomized controlled Norwegian study, researchers assessed the effect on twenty-seven patients with RA of a seven- to ten-day modified fast including vegetable juices and broths, followed by a lacto-vegetarian diet. A control group of twenty-six patients staying for four weeks at a convalescent home ate an ordinary diet throughout the study period. After four weeks at the health farm, the diet group showed a significant improvement in various objective and subjective indices of joint disease and pain: number of tender joints, Ritchie's articular index, number of swollen joints, pain score, duration of morning stiffness, grip strength, erythrocyte sedimentation rate, C-reactive protein, white blood cell count, and a health assessment questionnaire score. In the control group, none of these indices except pain score improved significantly. The diet group remained on a lacto-vegetarian diet for a year. The benefits of the diet were still present after that time, and evaluation of the whole course showed significant advantages for the group in all measured indices.[5] The dietary protocol for this study is discussed in chapter 13.

Earlier naturopathic reports included those of Dr. Herbert Shelton, who wrote that he had seen hundreds of cases of arthritis either cured or substantially relieved by fasting; and Dr. Paavo Airola, who reported similar results.[6] Both were writing in the 1960s and early 1970s.

DR. SHELTON'S OBSERVATIONS

Dr. Shelton asserted that "focal infections" (abscessed teeth, acute illness, emotional trauma, indigestion, colds, and other crises) could prompt an arthritic attack. But he maintained they are only secondary causes, the "last straw" that precipitates a crisis after the system has been weakened and resistance has been lowered by an accumulation of toxins at a faster rate than the body can metabolize them. The calcium deposits and stone formation that characterize arthritis point to an underlying nutritional problem—the same problem that causes the formation of gallstones and kidney stones, hardening of the arteries, deposits of lime on the valves of the heart, deposits in the feet in gout, and stone formation elsewhere in the body. Removing the secondary cause (for example, by pulling abscessed teeth) can alleviate the problem temporarily. But for a lasting cure, the body's toxic lode has to first be eliminated. If the arthritic condition is caught before permanent damage results, Dr. Shelton stated that fasting can not only relieve the pain but reverse the damage it has caused. The fast has to be followed by a fairly radical change in eating habits, however, to maintain its beneficial results.[7]

PRINCIPLES AND PROTOCOLS

Dr. Airola explained that after the first three days of fasting, your body lives on itself, burning and digesting its own tissues. However, it eliminates the dispensable ones first. That means that diseased, aging, or dead cells; morbid accumulations; tumors; abscesses; and damaged tissues are the first to go. During that time, the faster loses his craving for food. But when the nonessential tissues have been exhausted and the body is reduced to eating its own essential tissue, hunger suddenly returns with a vengeance. This is considered the physiologically correct time to end the fast.[8]

Dr. Shelton conducted long fasts on water only, but Dr. Airola recommended fasting on vegetable and fruit juices, and that not for more than seven to ten days unless under medical supervision. When our air was pure, our water was clean, our food was free of pesticides and preservatives, and the remedies we took for illness were natural herbs, we could safely fast on water. But today our environment has become so polluted and our bodies so laden with drugs, pesticides, and industrial wastes that long water fasts can be dangerous. Cleansing can proceed so rapidly that the released toxins overwhelm the body. We can control the speed of elimination of toxins and facilitate the body's ability to move them out by taking supplements and fresh-squeezed juices during a fast. A three-day juice fast is considered quite safe when undertaken at home, and it can give noticeable relief from joint pain.

Many people avoid fasting because they get headaches and feel weak whenever they go without food for a few hours. But if they can go without food for a longer period of time, they will find that the headaches will pass and they will feel more energetic than before they quit eating. The headaches and weakness are therefore not caused by lack of food. Fasting experts say these symptoms come because when we refrain from food for a while, our bodies take the opportunity to go into detox mode and dump toxins. While these toxins are passing through the bloodstream, we reexperience them. This is called a healing crisis and can make us feel worse before we feel better, but it is actually a sign that good things are happening.

My own first one-week fast, done at a health resort on juices and sprouts, was admittedly a miserable experience. But afterward, I felt marvelous; and each fast got easier after that. I did seven seven-day juice fasts spaced seven weeks apart, a protocol recommended by Dr. Bernard Jensen in the fasting classic *Tissue Cleansing Through Bowel Management*.[9] Since then, I have gone on a number of short fasts and now look forward to them like a vacation. My mind clears and I experience states verging on the mystical. To get to that level of appreciation, however, I had to go through a long series of fasts to detox my body of the accumulated effects of bad diet, pharmaceutical drugs, and other toxic buildup.

Although Dr. Shelton advised fasting without enemas, Dr. Airola thought daily enemas were essential to speed the elimination of toxins. Pamela Serure, in *Three Days to Vitality*, also recommends what she calls the "E" word—enemas. She observes that people don't want to think about this cleansing technique until they try it. Then they find how satisfying and relieving the experience can be.[10]

Dr. Jensen advises the use of coffee enemas during the fast to stimulate the liver to release toxins. The fast he recommends adds supplements (chlorophyll, beet, etc.), psyllium (plant fiber), and liquid bentonite clay (a natural colloidal adsorbing solution) to the prescribed regime. If you want to undertake a fast, Dr. Jensen's and Pamela Serure's books are excellent guides.

SKIN BRUSHING

Another detox technique recommended by Dr. Jensen when fasting is skin brushing, something he says is essential for anyone who wears clothes. The skin is a major organ of elimination, and new skin is made continually. Skin brushing with a natural bristle brush removes the top layer, leaving fresh new skin underneath. Healthy uncovered skin should dispose of two pounds of waste acids daily; but the skin's elimination is hampered by garments, oils, lotions, and the buildup of dirt and chemicals. To open the pores for proper cleansing, we need to stimulate it manually. Skin brushing helps eliminate uric acid crystals, catarrh, and other acids from the body. Dr. Jensen recommends brushing the entire body except the face with a natural bristle brush with a long handle. Don't use a nylon or plastic bristle brush. Use it dry on arising before dressing or bathing. For the face, a special face brush may be used.[11]

SKIN BRUSHING AND THE NIACIN FLUSH

Skin brushing is a particularly satisfying endeavor in combination with a detox treatment known as the niacin flush, which causes a flushing and itchiness of the skin. When your skin is red as a beet, with toxins itching to surface, skin brushing is an erotic experience. The niacin flush is used to purge the body of the fat-soluble environmental pollutants and heavy metals we have to deal with today. Although fasting is an excellent regime for clearing the body of backed-up metabolic wastes, it fails to eliminate these toxic metals and chemicals, which are so new to evolution that the body has no mechanism for detoxifying them. High-dose niacin and its effects on arthritis are the subject of the next two chapters.

NINE

Niacin and Arthritis

The body has an amazing ability to heal itself. Only a few things impede that process: environmental chemicals, viruses, and heavy metals.

—STEPHEN EDELSON, M.D.,
director of the Environmental and Preventive
Health Center in Atlanta, Georgia (1997)[1]

Niacin (nicotinamide or vitamin B_3) is sold as a cheap over-the-counter vitamin supplement in health food stores. It is also sold in high doses as a prescription product to lower elevated cholesterol levels, a use for which it is well known and highly effective. Less well known is the remarkable effectiveness of high-dose niacin in relieving arthritis symptoms. Abram Hoffer, M.D., a Canadian physician, reports dramatic results with arthritis simply from giving 2,000 to 3,000 milligrams of vitamin B_3 daily, along with other vitamins.

Dr. Hoffer discovered these effects by accident, when he was treating schizophrenics and alcoholics with niacin in the 1950s. He got so many unsolicited reports of improvement in arthritis symptoms that he could no longer ignore this unsuspected benefit. He thought his discovery was original until another researcher, William Kaufman, M.D., alerted him to Dr.

Kaufman's own books on the subject. Published in the 1940s, they documented in painstaking detail the beneficial effects on osteoarthritis of niacinamide, a form of vitamin B_3 closely related to niacin.[2]

Like Dr. Hoffer, Dr. Kaufman had made this discovery by accident while using niacin for other conditions. Dr. Kaufman detailed the responses of thousands of arthritics to niacinamide and other vitamin therapies, not only through their own subjective reports of pain relief but by extensive testing of joint mobility, muscle strength, and other objective measures of improvement. He measured twenty separate joint ranges in his patients and combined these measures into what he called the joint range index. Improvements in his patients' joint range indices provided conclusive evidence that niacinamide was working to reduce not just the subjective perception of pain but objective measures of joint injury. It was not simply reducing inflammation the way aspirin or cortisone does. It was actually repairing damaged joint surfaces. Improvements in the sedimentation rate (an objective blood test of pathology) paralleled those in the joint range index. Other objective measures also improved.

Although the treatment did not work for all of his patients, it did help a full 70 percent of them. Even patients with rheumatoid arthritis were helped, although RA involves not just degenerative but allergic, immunologic, and glandular components. Dr. Kaufman observed that the complications of RA are always superimposed on degenerative changes in the joint cartilage, and that those changes can be helped by niacinamide. For the treatment to work, the diet had to be sufficient in protein and calories; damage to the joints could not be so bad as to be irreversible; and the joints could not be subjected to continued, repetitive injury that prevented them from healing. Improvements generally occurred within three months of the start of treatment. Some patients also needed thiamine, B_6, and B_{12}.

Although Dr. Kaufman's original work and interest was not arthritis, he considered his most important contribution to nutritional medicine to be the discovery that treatment with niacinamide will improve impaired joint mobility in most people. The treatment proved to be quite safe even when taken for decades. He cited the case of a woman who took niacinamide for joint dysfunction from the ages of fifty-two to seventy-two. By the third year her joint problems had totally disappeared, and she retained the joint flexibility of a fifteen-year-old girl for the next seventeen years and beyond. In patients who discontinued treatment, however, joint flexibility again degenerated. The treatment had to be maintained to be effective.[3]

Dr. Hoffer, too, reported on an impressive series of cases involving niacin treatment. In an article in the December 1997 *Townsend Letter for Doctors & Patients,* he discussed three of many cases from his practice in which arthritis symptoms were miraculously relieved by a simple high-dose vitamin B_3 program. One patient had had the disease only three and one-half years and had not yet been damaged by chronic disease. She completely recovered from her symptoms on a program involving one gram of niacin three times daily, two grams of ascorbic acid (vitamin C) three times daily, 200 micrograms of selenium twice daily, 250 milligrams (mg) of pyridoxine, and 220 mg of zinc gluconate. The other two patients had suffered worse damage (one had irreversible skeletal deformities, including fingers that were permanently clawlike and unusable), but both experienced significant pain relief from a high-dose program of niacinamide.[4]

Jonathan Wright, M.D., a Harvard-trained Washington State physician, also reports impressive results with niacinamide. He notes that the pioneering work of Dr. Kaufman and Dr. Hoffer has been largely ignored by the scientific community, apparently because it involves a mere vitamin, which is not a lucrative proposition for drug companies; and because it was preempted by steroids, which hit the market at about the same time. Steroids were considered *the* cure for arthritis, until their serious side effects and drawbacks became known.[5]

Dr. Wright reported that in his practice niacinamide has relieved pain but has not proven to be a cure. It may be significant that only Dr. Hoffer's patient on *true* niacin was cured. Niacinamide and niacin are both forms of vitamin B_3, but they have different molecular structures and biological activity. Niacin produces a flush or blush—a redness and itchiness to the skin—while niacinamide doesn't. This flush is conventionally considered niacin's worst "side effect," but it may actually be a key factor in the treatment's success. A primary means of eliminating heavy metals and toxic chemicals from the body is through the skin by sweating. High doses of niacin aid this process by dilating the capillaries. The blood vessels expand so that blood rushes to the surface of the skin, carrying toxins with it. The face turns red and the skin turns hot as the niacin flushes out toxins.

SUPPLEMENTATION THERAPY OR DETOX TREATMENT?

Dr. Kaufman attributed the dramatic improvements in joint dysfunction brought about by high-dose niacin to a widespread deficiency of the vitamin. But while many symptoms improved just by adding niacin in modest doses (50 to 100 mg three times daily), many other cases responded only at very high doses (1,500 to 4,000 mg daily in divided doses).[6] The Recommended Daily Allowance (RDA) for vitamin B_3 is only 20 mg per day (the amount necessary to prevent pellagra). The dosage used for therapeutic purposes may be two thousand times that amount. Arthritis patients could hardly be "deficient" to that extent in vitamin B_3. Something else must be going on. Arguably, high-dose niacin relieves joint pain not because arthritics are gravely deficient in it but because the niacin "flush" flushes toxins from the joints. It is a detox rather than a supplementation therapy.

A detox treatment known as the niacin flush is actually used in drug rehabilitation centers to eliminate toxic drug and chemical buildup from the body. The dramatic effects of this treatment were demonstrated in a California study published in *Medical Hypotheses.* The program, which combined exercise and sauna or sweat therapy with high doses of niacin, was followed daily for a period of three weeks. It involved twenty to thirty minutes of vigorous exercise (jogging, stationary bicycling, rowing), followed by thirty minutes in the sauna, a five-minute cooling-off period, then thirty more minutes in the sauna. Sauna times could be gradually increased to two hours. Niacin dosage began at 400 mg spread throughout the day. The dose was then increased gradually to as high as 6,000 mg, depending on tolerance. Participants experienced significant drops in blood pressure, improvements in vision, increases in IQ points, and lessening of the symptoms of a number of physical ailments, including not only arthritic conditions but asthma, allergy, migraine, and hypoglycemia. Participants also reported reexperiencing the smells and physical effects of drugs taken in the past.[7]

According to Dr. David Williams, who writes an informative monthly newsletter called "Alternatives," the *only* method currently available for aiding the body in eliminating fat-soluble chemical toxins is the niacin flush. Fasting is excellent for eliminating metabolic wastes, but animal studies have shown that it won't eliminate fat-soluble chemicals. While fasting breaks down fat cells, the chemical toxins stored in these cells simply move from the fat into the muscles. When food is again eaten, they move back into the fat tissue.[8] If arthritis is due to a buildup of toxic residue in the joints, a detox procedure like the niacin flush seems to be essential for its reversal. The rationale and protocol of the niacin flush, along with studies establishing its safety and effectiveness, are the subject of the next chapter.

TEN

Eliminating Foreign Chemical Buildup with the Niacin Flush

Health is a precious thing, and the only one, in truth, meriting that a man should lay out, not only his time, sweat, labor and goods, but also his life itself to obtain it.

—MONTAIGNE,
Essays (1580)

High-dose niacin has not been thoroughly studied as an arthritis remedy. However, it has been studied and used in two other contexts: in the detoxification of xenobiotics (chemicals foreign to the human system) and in the treatment of high cholesterol levels. Both uses demonstrate its safety and effectiveness in eliminating toxic buildup from the body. Its use as a detoxification technique combined with sauna (sweating) not only reinforces the findings of Drs. Hoffer and Kaufman that it can reverse joint disease but suggests the mechanism.

DETOXIFYING XENOBIOTICS

In a 1992 review of the xenobiotics problem, Zane Gard, M.D., et al., explained that some chemicals readily dissolve in water, while others dissolve only in oil bases. Oil-soluble chemicals therefore have a tendency to accumulate in fatty tissue.

Oil-soluble chemicals include those commonly found in drugs (legal and illegal), household chemicals, toxic waste dumps, cosmetics, dry cleaning products, and chemical toxins in food and water. They include petroleum-based and oil-soluble pesticides and chemicals with ominous names like hexachlorobenzene, hexachlorocyclohexane (lindane), residues of chlordane (heptachloroepoxide, oxychlordane, transnonachlor), DDT residues, PCBs (polychlorinated biphenyls), THC, PCP, and dioxin. The National Academy of Sciences reports that the average American consumes forty milligrams of pesticides annually from food alone. These xenobiotics tend to accumulate in lipid deposits and adipose tissue throughout the body. The body does not know what to do with them or have mechanisms for breaking down and eliminating them.[1]

The body preserves its internal balance through homeostatic mechanisms, including detoxification by liver enzymes and the production of antibodies by the immune system. When these mechanisms are thrown off by xenobiotic chemicals, the result is disease. In one sobering study comparing women with breast cancer to controls, the cancer patients had a 50 to 60 percent higher concentration of PCBs in their tissues, as well as elevated levels of DDT and DDE. Researchers also suspect links with other diseases.[2]

The struggle with chemical insults either from a single toxic exposure or a lifetime of low-level chemical buildup can lead to a weakening or total breakdown of the immune system and other biological systems. The result can be a heightened sensitivity or intolerance to a variety of environmental substances. When individual tolerance thresholds are surpassed, pathological reactions occur.

Gard, et al., note that while many detoxification programs are available for removing circulating toxins from the bowels and for removing calcium deposits and plaque from the blood vessels and arteries, few are successful in eliminating fat-stored chemicals. Fasting is effective in removing toxic bacteria and metabolic wastes but not fat-soluble xenobiotics. Intravenous chelation therapy with EDTA (discussed in chapter 26) will successfully remove heavy metal buildup, as well as blockages from the buildup of calcium, fat, and cholesterol; but it, too, does little to mobilize fat-stored toxins unless they are already in the vascular system. In order to eliminate toxins from the body, they must be freed first from fat storage sites and flushed out by perspiration, in bile, and through other excretory pathways. An effective detoxification program must also replace any good elements that are eliminated along with the bad. Programs found effective in achieving these ends include heat-stress protocols that induce sweating and use high-dose niacin to facilitate elimination through the skin. Two with established track records are the Hubbard Method of Detoxification, started in 1978 as part of the drug rehabilitation program of NARC-ANON and currently available through the Church of Scientology; and the BioToxic Reduction Program, involving hyperthermic chambers, massage, exercise, and therapeutic doses of specific nutritional supplements.

A report issued by the Foundation for Advancement in Science and Education titled "Evaluation of a Detoxification for Fat Stored Xenobiotics" concluded that the Hubbard Method of Detoxification is safe and effective, significantly reducing blood pressure and cholesterol levels and improving psychological and IQ scores. Symptoms including joint pain, back pain, bursitis, and fibromyositis have also been significantly reduced.

The BioToxic Reduction Program described by Dr. Gard involved exercise followed by a minimum of two hours daily in the sauna at 140 to 180 degrees F (with periodic dips in the pool); high doses of niacin to increase peripheral circulation, release toxins from body storage sites, and stimulate the liver; vegetable oil (15 milliliters daily) to replace the contaminated fat and aid in its elimination through the bowels; nutritional supplements (vitamins, minerals, trace elements, oil, amino acids); and regular testing and monitoring. Therapy was done seven days a week for at least two weeks. Completion time for the average case was about three weeks, although serious cases could take six weeks. The body continued to detoxify on its own over a period of four to nine months, when more improvement was typically seen. Laboratory evidence showed that the toxic lode was significantly reduced by the end of the first month.[3]

Gard et al. detailed several cases in which joint pain was relieved by the BioToxic Reduction Program. One involved a woman with lupus whose hands before treatment were painful, swollen, clawlike, and barely usable. After treatment, complete range of motion returned to all of her joints, with no inflammation or soreness. Another woman had severe arthritis of the knee and had been scheduled for a surgical knee replacement. After the first day on the detox program, her arthritic symptoms eased and she could ride a stationary bike. After three weeks on the program, she experienced full range of motion and freedom from pain. She no longer needed medication or surgery.[4]

CAUTIONS WHEN TAKING NIACIN

Gard et al. caution that high doses of niacin should be taken only with professional supervision, which is needed to monitor the body's response and to ensure that toxins are properly eliminated. They assert that if all aspects of the program are not followed, these toxins could reenter the system.

Administrators of the Hubbard Program warn that when the toxins are put into circulation, the body is liable to have cleansing reactions like those experienced on original exposure (nausea, headaches, etc.). The psychological effects of narcotics and anesthetics may also be reexperienced. For this reason, sauna time should be spent with a friend who can intervene in case of crises. Heatstroke must also be watched for. It is signaled by a sudden cessation of sweating. If heatstroke seems imminent, the person should cool off immediately with a cool shower and take fluids, salt, and potassium.

Dr. David Williams (editor of "Alternatives," a monthly newsletter with up-to-date research on safe and effective therapies) asserts that the sauna portion of the program may be done at your local health club, and that the niacin/sauna detoxification is "simple, inexpensive, and safe, as long as it is done under the supervision of your doctor." He observes that the high temperatures involved in sauna therapy put an extra burden on the heart and cardiovascular system, so you should check with your doctor to make sure you have no medical conditions that would make the program dangerous for you. The program should be started slowly and increased gradually as your body gets used to it. It should be followed for about three weeks. Specific nutritional supplements should also be taken to replace losses and allow the body to rebuild itself from healthy raw materials.

DR. WILLIAMS'S PROTOCOL

Here is the regimen Dr. Williams recommends:

Exercise for twenty to thirty minutes by jogging on a treadmill or using a stationary bicycle or rowing machine. Exercise triggers sweating, which starts the process of toxic elimination. Sweating, he observes, can release as much toxic material as elimination through the kidneys.

Sauna to maintain the sweating process. Begin with thirty minutes at 140 to 180 degrees followed by a five-minute cooling-off period, followed by another thirty minutes in the sauna. Over three or four days increase to two hours in the sauna if desired, with short cooling-off periods. Drink plenty of water in the sauna to avoid dehydration. (Hubbard administrators advise salt tablets. Solutions can also be purchased at health food stores to replace electrolytes.)

Niacin beginning at 400 mg daily, gradually increasing to about 3,000 mg daily. Dr. Williams suggests spreading the dose throughout the day. (In the Hubbard Program, by contrast, niacin is taken in a single dose with yogurt or some other food just before sweating is induced with exercise and sauna.)

Vitamin C in the range of 2,000 to 8,000 mg daily, spread throughout the day to avoid diarrhea. Vitamin C protects against cellular changes and altered enzyme activity that can result when toxins are released into the bloodstream for elimination.

Vitamin E: 400 to 800 International Units (IU) daily.

Vitamin A: 25,000 IU daily (or 15 mg of beta-carotene).

Calcium/magnesium supplement: one providing 1,000 mg of calcium and 500 mg of magnesium daily.

Multivitamin/mineral supplement: one containing not only the usual nutrients but a range of trace minerals including chromium, selenium, manganese, and zinc. It should also contain 50 mg of the major B-vitamins to balance niacin intake, since vitamins work synergistically with each other. If these are not sufficiently provided in the multivitamin/mineral supplement, a separate B-complex vitamin pill should be taken.

Flaxseed oil: one to two tablespoons daily.

Lecithin: two tablespoons daily, to help remove DDT metabolites that may be released into the bloodstream.

Additional vitamins, minerals, amino acids, and fatty acids may be required by some people. This can be determined through urine and blood evaluations by your doctor.[5]

ANOTHER LOOK AT THE SAFETY ISSUE:
THE EVIDENCE FROM CONVENTIONAL
HYPERLIPIDEMIA TREATMENT

Confirming the safety of high-dose niacin is its well-documented use as a remedy for lowering elevated cholesterol levels. Niacin is the oldest and most versatile agent used in the treatment of hyperlipidemia (elevated concentrations of lipids in the blood plasma). In that context, it has an established track record not only for cholesterol-lowering benefits leading to a proven reduction in coronary artery disease incidence, but for safety and effectiveness for most people even when taken in high doses over long periods.[6] Note that for arthritis, the niacin flush is not proposed for long periods. Three weeks is usually sufficient to remove toxic accumulations from the joints.

The Coronary Drug Project, involving 8,000 people over a six-year period, showed that niacin can be taken for years with only minor side effects. Robert Kowalski, in a bestselling book called *The 8-Week Cholesterol Cure,* states that most people can reach the level of 3,000 mg daily without side effects. But he still advises checking with your doctor first, since people with impaired liver function, gout, elevated uric acid levels, ulcers, or diabetes could be at risk. Kowalski's recommended protocol is to begin with 100 mg of niacin three times daily, increasing every third day to the therapeutic dose. For lowering cholesterol levels, he recommends a pharmaceutical version of niacin called "Endur-acin," which can give the same or better therapeutic effect at half the dose, thus reducing niacin's main "side effect," the flush.[7]

To avoid the flush, researchers have also tried using time-release niacin; but further study has shown this pharmaceutical product to have worse drawbacks than the flush. In a 1991 study, inflammation of the liver developed in five patients who were taking relatively low dosages (three grams per day or less) of the time-release form; and in four of the five patients, clinical symptoms of hepatitis developed after the medication had been taken for a fairly short time (two days to seven weeks). This differed from earlier reports of liver problems in conjunction with crystalline niacin, which had occurred only with quite high dosage after prolonged use.[8] In 1992, *The American Journal of Medicine* also reported that hepatic toxicity occurred more frequently with time-release preparations than with unmodified niacin.[9]

Again, the flush may not be a "side effect" but may be the very mechanism by which niacin succeeds in cleaning out the system. Toxins accumulate not only in the arteries, raising cholesterol levels, but in the joints, causing arthritic pain. The conventional theory attributes elevated blood cholesterol levels to excess dietary cholesterol. An alternative hypothesis, however, is that blood cholesterol levels become elevated because the body pads its arteries with cholesterol to protect them from onslaughts by toxins. Niacin works on both arthritis and elevated cholesterol levels by increasing circulation, thus helping to eliminate accumulated toxins. Flushing indicates that the niacin is pushing toxic substances to the surface of the skin.

Other possible side effects reported for high-dose niacin include gastrointestinal discomfort and, in rare cases after prolonged usage, liver toxicity. The latter evidently results when the released toxins build up in the liver faster than they can be eliminated. For this reason people with impaired liver function should not undertake a niacin flush; but for people with adequate liver function, the problem can be avoided and the flush can be relieved by accompanying the procedure with other detox measures designed to speed the process, including sauna, exercise, sweating, and a full nutritional supplement program. Discomfort from the flush can also be reduced by starting at a low dose and working up. As the body releases its toxins, uncomfortable flushing occurs only at higher and higher doses.

A friend who went through the Hubbard Program to eliminate drug toxicity acquired from a long hospital stay reported that 100 mg of niacin was actually more uncomfortable for him than 5,000 mg. This was because he worked into it gradually, using the other Hubbard techniques along with the niacin to speed elimination. He reported coming away from the program feeling "reborn" and "like a child again."

For people who find the flush too daunting, niacin's flush-free molecular cousin niacinamide remains a good option. Although niacinamide doesn't work for lowering cholesterol, Dr. Hoffer and Dr. Kaufman both reported beneficial results on arthritic symptoms with its use. Niacinamide may, in fact, work on arthritis by a different mechanism than forcing toxins out through the skin. Dr. Kaufman found that frequency of dosing was important. Niacinamide breaks down in the body relatively quickly. Joint range index measurements indicated that 250 mg every three hours worked better than 500 mg every six hours. Recommended intake ranged from 900 to 4,000 mg daily, divided into from six to sixteen doses.

PERSONAL EXPERIENCE

My own home niacin protocol was devised by trial and error based on a study I had read. I did a three-week flush, during which I got up to a daily dose of 2,000 mg. I then dropped back down to 1,000 mg (taken in a single dose), which seemed to be quite effective for me. I did this program without professional supervision, but I was healthy except for an ailing hip. I tempered the flush by using other detox procedures that aided the process of drawing out toxins and eliminating them, including skin brushing, clay poultices (discussed in the next chapter), and homeopathic detox remedies (discussed in chapter 27).

As soon as I began that course of treatment, my hip quit bothering me at night and I began to sleep well. By the end of three weeks, I noticed no symptoms at all, until nine months later when I overstressed my hip. Now I take 500 mg of niacin whenever I feel like a good pore-cleanse. I follow it with twenty or thirty minutes on the treadmill and an hour in the sauna, accompanied by skin brushing. If the sun is out, I then indulge in a sunbath. When the pores are open and clean, the kiss of the sun is bliss.

ELEVEN

The Remarkable Properties of Clay

How can a natural remedy as simple and cheap as clay perform such complex actions as: to void an abscess, to heal a sore, rebuild a vertebral column, reabsorb a cyst (even internal), relocate a badly placed foetus, help to rebuild destroyed tissue? . . . We were so astounded with each new result, and results were so often beyond expectation, that we realized clay has many more healing possibilities which are as yet unexplored.

—DR. RAYMOND DEXTREIT,
Our Earth Our Cure (1974)[1]

Raymond Dextreit, a French naturopathic doctor, relates the remarkable case of a man who was saved from hip surgery by clay poultices. The man was only thirty-seven when he had his first arthritic attack. His doctors' solution was to operate. Instead, the patient used the naturopathic technique of applying nightly clay poultices to the affected hip, and his pain gradually went away. When he returned for an X ray many months later, his arthritis had disappeared. His doctors could not explain this unprecedented phenomenon. Their only suggestion was that his X rays and prior examinations must have been in error.

Clay poultices?! How could the simple application of mud

packs cure an arthritic hip? Dextreit starts with the naturopathic explanation for the disease: arthritis results when toxic
substances accumulate around the joints and obstruct the capillaries. This causes an accumulation of residues of metabolic
wastes—crystals of sodium urate, uric or oxalic acid, and so
on—which hinder the entrance of oxygen and food elements to
the site. The result is inflammation, then lesions of the cartilage
and later of the bone. A fibrous tissue eventually replaces the
destroyed cartilage, limiting movement. The limited motion,
fibrous thickening, and fluid accumulation strain the joints and
create pain. Clay poultices relieve this pain by drawing out and
removing toxic substances from the body.

Mud has long been known for its therapeutic properties.
Mudpacks and mud baths are popular therapies used worldwide
for detoxification, skin cleansing, and pain relief. If you have
ever had a full-body mud bath in a spa, you know how absolutely rejuvenating this therapy can be. Why? Mud and clay
have the remarkable property of attracting and absorbing toxins
and harmful bacteria. Clay is an *"ad*sorbent"—an agent that at-
tracts other materials or particles to its surface. Everything emit-
ting unhealthy negative radiations, says Dextreit, is irresistibly
attracted to clay's positive pole and becomes subject to immediate elimination.

MEDICAL STUDIES ON CLAY

Dextreit's claims concerning clay's toxin-removing abilities are
confirmed by studies from medical journals. Here are a few:

Sodium bentonite (montmorillonite), a form of clay used
commercially in foundries to hold sand and water together to
form a mold for molten metal, was investigated in a Norwegian
study in which the feed of dairy cattle was treated with bentonite after the Chernobyl accident. The researchers reported

that elevated radiocaesium levels in the feed were successfully reduced.[2]

In a Tennessee study, thirteen mice were injected with blood plasma from a human patient with a fatal form of pneumonia. All thirteen mice died within twelve hours. When the blood plasma was first treated with an adsorbing product including clay, no deaths occurred in thirteen of another set of thirteen mice after twelve hours. The bacterial toxins contained in the plasma had been detoxified by adsorption.[3]

In a Pennsylvania study, a skin lotion containing bentonite clay was found to be effective in preventing or diminishing experimentally produced allergic contact dermatitis from poison ivy and poison oak in 144 subjects having a history of poison oak or poison ivy allergy. The researchers noted that clay applied externally has healing properties, and that natural mud baths are a well-known folk remedy for arthritic pains.[4]

Italian researchers found that a skin product containing bentonite clay had remarkable therapeutic value in the treatment of skin wounds and burns. The product was well tolerated, and healing occurred without scars.[5]

Bentonite clay and another mineral soil called "Fuller's earth" are both used conventionally in the treatment of paraquat poisoning. In a European study, researchers observed that the curative effect of these clays results from their ability to absorb poison.[6]

Researchers at the University of Kentucky investigating geophagia, the eating of dirt (usually clay), noted that this practice has been recorded in every region of the world, and that in some societies it is culturally endorsed. Although conventionally considered pathological, the researchers concluded that the practice has health benefits, since clay detoxifies and acts as an antidiarrheal and a source of minerals.[7]

THE HISTORY OF CLAY THERAPY

The therapeutic uses of clay have actually been known for thousands of years. The Egyptians were aware of its purifying powers and used it to mummify their dead. Greek physicians, including Dioscorides and Galen, knew of it and used it. Pliny the Elder, a first-century Roman naturalist, devoted an entire chapter of his *Natural History* to it. "Primitive" tribes around the world not only use clay externally but take it internally. In India, Mahatma Gandhi advised its use. In Europe, the therapeutic application of clay was revived by the great nineteenth-century German naturopaths Kneipp, Kuhn, Just, and Felke. "Luvos" earth, a remedy developed by Adolph Just, is still used.

In a remarkable 1904 book called *Return to Nature,* Dr. Just reported curing a broad range of conditions that were otherwise considered incurable, including arthritis, using only the tools of nature. His protocol included applying clay poultices, sleeping naked directly on the ground (covered by a woolen blanket), taking sunbaths and cold water hip baths (described in chapter 21), and eating a diet consisting of fruits, nuts, raw milk, butter, and a little bread. One patient described by Dr. Just had suffered from chronic inflammatory rheumatoid arthritis for a number of years. He was quite paralyzed and had reached the dire stage of requiring a leg amputation when he learned of Dr. Just's treatment. Using the doctor's natural therapies, the patient avoided loss of his leg.[8]

In a 1994 book called *More Precious than Gold,* researcher Ray Pendergrast reports that a form of calcium bentonite clay called Pascalite has saved gangrenous legs from amputation, along with reversing many other conditions including arthritis.[9]

PERSONAL EXPERIENCE

I'll add a personal anecdote involving leg amputation. The young son of my housekeeper's cousin in Nicaragua had a very badly infected leg. He was on antibiotics, but the drugs were making him sick and the leg just kept getting worse. The doctor said that if the antibiotics did not work, the leg would have to be amputated. I gave my housekeeper a five-pound bag of bentonite clay ($1.50 at the local Nicaraguan health food store) and told her how to make clay poultices with it. Two weeks later she reported that, "Gracias a Dios," the child's leg had healed. The doctor could not believe it and asked the mother what she had done. When she showed him the bag of clay, he remained baffled but said to keep it up, as it was working.

Clay poultices also brought noticeable improvement to my own arthritic hip. I did two three-week series of them, spaced six months apart. The first series brought about sufficient improvement that I was convinced the therapy worked, but it was the second series that struck me as remarkable. By then I had essentially lost interest in my hip, which hardly bothered me. Far more interesting were the changes in my energy level and sense of overall well-being. I was, I felt, growing younger.

You can convince yourself of the therapeutic benefits of dirt in fifteen minutes by visiting a natural mud spa. I took a full-body mud bath at a spa in Calistoga, in Northern California, at a time when I was particularly stressed, was having trouble sleeping, and ached in my muscles and joints. The fifteen-minute mud bath was followed by a hot bath in mineral water, a steam bath, and a massage. That night I slept like a baby and awoke refreshed and pain-free.

Clay not only is a great natural remedy that effects remarkable rejuvenation of the body but is "dirt" cheap. It can actually be dug from your garden (clays from your local area are considered the most "sympathetic"), but health food stores provide bentonite clay in neatly packaged powders and liquids that are more convenient. Clay may be used externally or internally. Internal use is easier but external poultice applications treat specific areas more directly. They are also a fascinating exercise in healing. That something so ubiquitous as mud (or urine) could have rejuvenating properties suggests that the solution to the health care crisis could be right beneath our feet.

PROTOCOL FOR USING CLAY POULTICES

For treating arthritis, Dextreit states that clay poultices should be used daily. Regardless of the ultimate body part to be treated, they should be applied first to the lower abdomen, where all poultice treatment begins. Then they are placed on the site of the affected joint. In my case, I applied poultices for a week to the lower abdomen, then for two more weeks to my arthritic hip.

To make clay poultices for external application, half fill a large, deep bowl with powdered bentonite clay. Then cover with unboiled water, so that the water comes to approximately half an inch over the clay. Don't mix; mixed clay loses its porosity and becomes smooth and impermeable. Place the bowl in the sun or open air for an hour or so, covering with a gauze to avoid impurities. Clay, says Dextreit, picks up and transmits radiations from the earth and atmosphere. The more it is exposed to sun, rain and air, the more active it becomes. Let the clay sit for several hours and absorb the water on its own.

When preparing clay, do not leave it in contact with metal or plastic spoons or bowls, from which it can draw unwanted chemicals. Instead use wood, ceramics, glass, porcelain, or earthenware. Powdered clay may, however, be stored in a plastic container.

Poultices can be prepared in various ways. I did it by placing a folded paper towel on two folded washcloths, which were placed on a strip of cotton cloth large enough to be tied around my abdomen. I ladled the moist clay onto the paper towel, without spreading or stirring. If the mud mixture was too thin to stay in place, I added some powdered clay to thicken; if it was too thick to be comfortable, I added some water. Then I tied the whole contraption around my abdomen, with the clay pressed directly to my skin. Different thicknesses of mud are recommended for different conditions, but for an arthritic hip, a patty about an inch thick and covering as much of the hip as possible is recommended. The initial poultices to the lower abdomen should also be about one inch thick and should cover a wide area.

Various means of attaching a poultice to the body may be used, including tying it on with a wide strip of cloth, wrapping it in ace bandages, or, if the area to be covered is hard to encircle, by taping it on with bandages. The clay should touch the body and can be pressed in place to cover the entire area. Apply poultices once a day (no more) for ninety minutes to four hours, well spaced between meals. For the stomach area, the application of poultices needs to be completely out of the digestive period, at least two hours after the last meal and an hour before the next one. Don't do lower-abdomen poultices if you are menstruating. Poultices can be left on overnight, but if they become uncomfortable or make you cold, take them off. For acute pain, as in gout, they may be applied one after the other to the affected area, each one remaining in place for two to three hours.

As with fasting, your symptoms may get worse before they get better; but this is actually a good sign. It means the clay is doing its job of drawing toxins out of the body. As they pass through the treated area, the area is likely to feel more symptomatic. But this soon passes, and in the end you'll feel significantly better than when you started.

Dextreit stated that the length of treatment varies with the case, but that it should be kept up until disappearance of the problem. He warned not to interrupt a clay series once begun, since clay starts a cleansing process throughout the organism that could do more harm than good if terminated before completion. Toxins drawn halfway out could be more uncomfortable than those left buried in the tissues. Even when the series is finished, he said, clay should be discontinued gradually, from every day to twice a week to once a week. (That was his warning, but I was rather erratic in my clay experiments without noticeable mishap.)

Clay should not be applied to more than one site at a time and should not be painful or uncomfortable. Unlikely but possible side effects are red patches and intense itching resulting from acid substances passing from internal organs. If these occur, said Dr. Dextreit, the poultices should be discontinued.

Clay should be thrown away after use and not touched, since it now contains toxic substances. The cloths used to attach it may be washed and reused, however. Clay use should not be combined with medicines, whether conventional or homeopathic, since the medicines inhibit its action. If drugs must be taken, however, external clay treatment is less affected by them than internal clay treatment.

Those cautions aside, Dextreit asserted that clay is quite safe and that there is no reason not to give it a try. In every case, he observed remarkable improvement; and in some cases, complete healing. He recommended giving the poultice treatment a three- or four-month trial before abandoning it.

ORAL CLAY TREATMENT

Clay can also be taken orally. Dextreit's suggested oral usage for adults is to put a teaspoon of powdered clay in half a glass of un-boiled water. Clay works not by supplying missing nutrients but by a catalytic action, so a teaspoon is all you need. Taking more won't increase its activity and could upset your system. If possible, prepare the clay several hours earlier or the night before use, and drink it on arising or at bedtime. It should be taken at least fifteen to twenty minutes before eating, although an hour is better. Taken before food, it will sedate stomach pains after the meal but can also slow up the bowels. If the opposite effect is desired, take it before bed. Use it for three weeks, then alternate one week on and one week off.

The product recommended for adsorbing toxins by Dr. Bernard Jensen, author of a number of popular books on fasting and naturopathy, is a bentonite clay called "Sonne's No. 7," which comes bottled in liquid form. The adult dosage suggested on the label is one tablespoonful twice daily, the first in warm water on arising and the other undiluted at the time of the evening meal. Drinking at least one glass of water between meals is also advised, to assist elimination of acid and toxic waste through the kidneys.[10]

Pascalite is another form of bentonite clay reported to heal a wide range of conditions including arthritis. Pascalite is calcium bentonite, a form with less industrial value than sodium bentonite but significant therapeutic value. In my own case, a mere quarter teaspoon taken daily in juice on an empty stomach not only had a beneficial effect on my joints but boosted my energy level. The product is available from Pascalite, Inc., P.O. Box 104, Worland, Wyoming 82401; telephone 307-347-3872.

SUPPLEMENTARY THERAPIES

Other treatments Dr. Dextreit recommends for arthritis include cold hip baths (discussed in chapter 21), sunbaths, and herbs to activate elimination. (Herbal laxative products are available at health food stores.) He suggests that clay treatment be preceded by at least ten days of a natural purifying vegetarian diet, laxative teas, and a lemon treatment to reduce the toxic load of the body (half a lemon in 4 to 8 ounces of hot or cold water, with honey if desired, one or more times daily). For general tonic and detox-ification purposes, the following drinks are recommended in the morning on an empty stomach:

Week 1: Take a teaspoon of powdered clay in half a glass of water, prepared the night before. Alternatively, use a tablespoon of a commercial liquid bentonite preparation, which needn't be specially prepared.

Week 2: Mix a teaspoon of olive oil with an equal amount of lemon juice and drink it before breakfast. Dextreit observed that olive oil is an excellent natural laxative and stimulates the secre-tion of the juices of the liver and pancreas; and that lemon also stimulates, decongests, and cleanses the liver, as well as dissolv-ing and eliminating crystallized toxins lodged in the joints.

Alternate these treatments for one month. Then three times a week substitute for the olive oil–lemon juice mixture an eggshell–lemon juice concoction, prepared as follows:

In the evening, put a whole egg with its shell, well cleaned, into a cup and cover with lemon juice. Let soften overnight. In the morning, remove the egg, which can be used for cooking purposes; then drink the liquid. The calcium absorbed from the shell will aid in recalcifying the joint bones by stimulating the assimilation and fixation of calcium in the body.

For a lasting cure, Dextreit stresses that dietary change is es-sential. That therapeutic tool is the subject of the next chapter.

TWELVE

The Role of Diet and Digestion

I am convinced digestion is the great secret of life.

—REV. SYDNEY SMITH,
Works (1859)

To Dr. Dextreit, as to Dr. Shelton, the underlying problem in arthritis is nutritional. Dextreit attributes arthritic and rheumatic disorders of all types to the same degenerative process: the buildup in the blood of metabolic wastes and other toxic substances, including urea, uric acid, cholesterol, acetone, ammonia, and phosphates. These cause the blood to thicken, the circulation to slow, the tissues to become asphyxiated from lack of oxygen, and the muscles to contract. The result is rheumatic and arthritic pain. The accumulation of residues of metabolic wastes around the joints hinders the entrance of food and oxygen, causing an inflammatory condition, then lesions of the cartilage and later of the bone. The body replaces what is lost with a fibrous tissue that limits movement of the joints. The tendons may also calcify and lose their flexibility. Although "wear and tear" localizes the symptoms, the underlying problem is wrong diet and absorption of toxins.

A diet high in nitrogenous meats and proteins, along with other acids that come directly from food, combines with the acidic residues of muscular activity, causing acidic wastes to pre-dominate. Meat causes calcium (an alkaline mineral) to be pulled from the bones as a buffer. Natural sulfur is also required to neutralize the poisons resulting from digestion. Indol, one of the degradation products of animal cells, requires an enormous amount of sulfur for neutralization. Since sulfur is also necessary for the fixation of calcium, using the body's sulfur stores for neutralizing animal products is disastrous for calcification of the bones.

Compounding the problem are drugs that wipe out friendly intestinal bacteria that destroy uric acid and other metabolic wastes. These drugs include not only antibiotics, which kill friendly and unfriendly bacteria indiscriminately, but most of the drugs prescribed for arthritic conditions. Aspirin prevents the reproduction of bacteria, including those that detoxify uric acid. So do cortisone and its derivatives, which have many other harmful effects as well. Antiseptics and certain chemicals in commercial foods can also destroy beneficial bacteria.

To cure these conditions permanently, not only should drugs be avoided but the diet must be changed. Dr. Dextreit recom-mends an essentially vegan diet, supplemented with yogurt and buttermilk and emphasizing raw food (fruit and vegetables) and cereals (sprouted wheat, whole wheat bread, hulled barley, brown rice, couscous, millet, oats, rye, buckwheat). He also warns to stay away from foods generating acids or containing acidifying poisons, including alcohol and alkaloids—especially coffee. (If, like me, you absolutely can't give up coffee, a com-promise solution is to drink an acid-free caffeinated coffee sold under the brand name Kava. Better yet is green tea, which con-tains caffeine but in smaller amounts and has joint-friendly anti-inflammatory properties.)

Even after the diet is changed to a healthy one, says Dextreit, eliminating metabolic wastes is a lengthy process. He recommends garlic and cabbage to help replenish sulfur stores, and fresh vegetable juices (carrot, cabbage, turnip, etc.) to provide the elements necessary for rebuilding the joints. Juicing allows the ingestion of large quantities of nutrients without chewing great quantities of vegetables.

RESEARCH ESTABLISHING
THE DIETARY CONNECTION

In the 1980s, the Arthritis Foundation asserted categorically that there is no special diet for arthritis; that no specific food has anything to do with causing it; and that no specific diet will cure it. But few researchers today question the likelihood of a dietary component to the disease, and many recent studies have shown a link. There are foods and nutritional supplements that help the condition, and foods and additives that make it worse. There are also effective supplementation therapies that work by addressing nutritional deficiencies.

Studies showing a link with nutrition first appeared for rheumatoid arthritis. Several studies published in the 1980s associated RA with food intolerances. One published in the *Annals of Internal Medicine* in 1987 showed that about 5 to 10 percent of all cases of RA were due to food intolerances. In another double-blind study, patients with RA were first fed a two-week wash-out diet of foods unlikely to cause allergic reactions. Then they were challenged with capsules of either placebos or known food allergens—dairy products, wheat, corn, citrus, coffee, and chocolate—to determine the foods to which they were sensitive. The effect of different foods was very individual, but about 15 percent of subjects improved dramatically and 70 percent showed varying degrees of improvement so long as the particular foods to which they were intolerant were not in their diets.[1]

Other studies have been done with mice. Laboratory studies have shown that underfeeding and a low-caloric diet reduce the spontaneous development of osteoarthritis in mice, whereas a high-caloric diet promotes the disease. In man, mice, and fattened animals, obesity is often associated with forms of osteoarthritis.[2] Weight loss is routinely recommended for overweight people with the disease, since carrying around an extra fifty pounds or so adds an unnatural burden to the weight-bearing joints. A thick layer of fat between the tendons and ligaments can also separate them so the joints no longer function correctly mechanically.[3]

ARTHRITIS AND DIETARY FAT

Still other studies link arthritis to dietary fat. In one, complete remissions resulted in six patients with rheumatoid arthritis when they changed to a fat-free diet. Symptoms returned within three days of ingesting fat, whether in the form of animal fat or vegetable oils. The researchers concluded that dietary fats in amounts normally eaten can cause the inflammatory joint changes seen in rheumatoid arthritis.[4]

Researchers at Wayne State University in Detroit documented the cases of two obese RA patients who were put on a strict low-fat diet. Symptoms disappeared after only five days and were absent for more than a year. Lawrence Power, M.D., who helped develop the diet, explained that the body needs fat to produce the prostaglandins that fuel inflammation. Without this fuel, the inflammation subsides. The culprit was found to be not animal fat or any other particular fat but fat in general. After making this discovery, the researchers worked with thirty RA patients and found that nine out of ten of them experienced relief by cutting fat from their diets.

In the 1970s, Nathan Pritikin reported similar results with

patients with osteoarthritis, following the stringent low-fat diet recommended at his Longevity Center in Santa Monica, California. One dramatic case involved an eighty-one-year-old woman who had such severe arthritis in her knee that she could not walk up stairs. After a year on the Pritikin diet, her joint function returned. After four years on it, at the age of eighty-five, she won two gold medals in a Senior Olympics, one for the mile race and the other for the half mile.

Like the Wayne State University researchers, Pritikin thought fat itself was the culprit in RA. It was not even a matter of being overweight, just of eating too much fat. Fat reduces circulation by coating the red blood cells, preventing them from passing through the small blood vessels. Oxygen levels then drop and the immune system is weakened, allowing powerful enzymes to leak into the joint, resulting in RA. Pritikin considered salt to be another culprit, since it causes the tissues to be flooded with water, also reducing circulation. For people with arthritic knees and hips, his program reportedly worked on half of them; and for people with arthritic hands, fingers, and wrists, it worked on 90 percent of them.[5]

THE "GOOD" FATS

That research aside, some types of fat have been found to be good for arthritic joints. Scientists first discovered the benefits of the fatty acids in fish oils in the 1970s, when Danish physicians observed that Greenland Eskimos had very little arthritis and heart disease although they ate a high-fat animal foods diet. Most animal foods contain omega-6 fats, which increase the inflammatory response of the body; but the omega-3 fatty acids found in fish enable the body to make the products it needs to decrease this response. The most commonly available omega-3 fatty acid is EPA (eicosapentaenoic acid), found in some fish and fish oil. EPA capsules are also available in health food stores. Studies show that eating high-fat fish containing omega-3 fatty acids (including mackerel, bluefish, tuna, herring, anchovies, sardines, and salmon) helps decrease the inflammation of arthritis.[6]

Both seafood and unrefined vegetable oils contain linoleic and alpha linolenic acids. These are the "essential fatty acids" (EFAs) that cannot be made by the human body but must be ingested in the diet. EFAs are grouped into two families, omega-6 EFAs and omega-3 EFAs. Both are necessary, but they need to be in balance. We evolved on a diet containing roughly equal amounts of omega-3 and omega-6 fatty acids, but commercialization and dietary change has skewed this percentage so that it is now about 20 or 25 to one in favor of the omega-6 fatty acids.

In part, this shift was due to the hydrogenation of vegetable oil, which turned it from an unsaturated to a saturated fat. Fats are "saturated" when their carbon atoms are linked to as many hydrogen atoms as they can hold. "Unsaturated" fats, which can absorb more hydrogen, are liquid at room temperature. Hydrogenation, or adding hydrogen, turns liquid oils to solids at room temperature (as in margarine or shortening) by "saturating" the carbon openings with hydrogen.

Many of the beneficial effects of a diet rich in plant foods are the result of its low levels of saturated fat and relatively higher levels of EFAs. A diet high in saturated fat has been linked to many chronic diseases, while a diet low in saturated fat but high in EFAs has been found to prevent the same diseases.[7] Increasing the intake of EFAs over an extended period of time has also been shown to decrease the pain, inflammation, and limitation of motion of arthritic joints.[8]

Cold-pressed polyunsaturated fats (safflower, sunflower, corn, and other vegetable oils) contain both omega-6 and omega-3 EFAs. Omega-3 is most abundant in flaxseed oil, but soy, pumpkin seed, evening primrose, borage seed, walnut, and black currant seed oils are also good sources.[9]

ARTHRITIS AND SUGAR

Along with the "bad" fats, sugar and refined carbohydrates are high on the list of dietary hazards for arthritics. Overindulgence in sugar can accelerate joint deterioration by exhausting calcium stores, thus weakening bone structure. The breakdown products of sugar are acidic, requiring calcium (a base) to buffer them. Excess sugar can also stimulate or aggravate arthritis by inducing hypoglycemia (low blood sugar), a common symptom of which is joint pain. Other symptoms include numbness, leg cramps, twitching and jerking of leg muscles, restlessness, irritability, depression, anxiety, and phobias. The emotional brain is extremely sensitive to drops in blood sugar. These symptoms have been observed to disappear when the hypoglycemia was brought under control. Even cases diagnosed as rheumatoid arthritis have cleared up when the patients' hypoglycemia was resolved. Disturbances of starch-sugar metabolism are particularly common in rheumatoid arthritics.

A too-quick rise in blood sugar can result not only from sugar consumption but from caffeine intake, since caffeine stimulates the adrenal glands to produce hormones that raise blood sugar. The body responds by producing insulin to burn off the excess glucose. An excess insulin response then lowers the blood sugar. Eating sugar causes the blood sugar to shoot up, then precipitously fall, prompting you to crave more sugar. To break the sugar habit, the best approach is to simply quit eating sugar. You crave it because you indulge in it rather than the reverse.[10]

THE ENZYME FACTOR

Almost two-thirds of the calories most people eat consist of fat and refined carbohydrates (sugar, white flour products, and the like). As we continue to eat these nutrient-deficient foods along with foods that are frozen, canned, processed, and overcooked, we become increasingly deficient not only in essential vitamins and minerals but in enzymes, because cooking, microwaving, and processing destroy the enzymes found naturally in foods. That means the nutrients we do get in our food aren't properly absorbed, since our food lacks the enzymes necessary to digest them.

Enzymes and hydrochloric acid in the stomach break down protein and fat, enhance mineral absorption, and aid digestion. Enzymes from the pancreas then divide fats, protein, and carbohydrates down further in the small intestine and prepare them for absorption. To replace the enzymes lost in cooking, the pancreas must work overtime to make pancreatic enzymes; and to overcome the inhibitory effects of fat on sugar utilization, the pancreas must make extra insulin. The liver, which metabolizes carbohydrates and makes the bile necessary for fat digestion, also gets overworked. Supplemental vitamins, minerals, digestive enzymes, and antioxidants may be taken in pill form, but to attack the problem at its roots requires changing the diet to one of whole, unprocessed, largely raw food.[11]

GENERAL DIETARY RECOMMENDATIONS

The first step in joint-healthy nutrition is to eliminate junk food from the diet—including candy, pastries, soft drinks, and white-flour products such as spaghetti, macaroni, noodles, and white bread. The best foods for arthritics are whole foods—

fruits, vegetables, grains, nuts, and cold water fish. "Good" oils are also essential. The omega-3 fats found in vegetables and fish help nourish joint tissue. The omega-6 fats found in beef, pork, and poultry, on the other hand, produce prostaglandins that can increase the level of inflammation in the joints. Alcohol should be avoided, since it can deplete the body of magnesium and other joint-protective nutrients and can impair the liver, thus interfering with proper cartilage formation. Other foods that arthritis specialists recommend cutting down on or omitting include eggs, margarine, shortening, and dairy products, all of which contain saturated fat.

Other foods may need to be avoided because of individual sensitivities to them. That factor is discussed next.

THIRTEEN

Arthritis, Food Allergies, and Toxic Foods

> *Now good digestion wait on appetite,*
> *And health on both!*
>
> —SHAKESPEARE, *Macbeth*

In *How to Eat Away Arthritis,* Dr. Lauri Aesoph suggests that the reason nutrition has been downplayed as a cause of the disease is that no single diet works for every arthritis sufferer. The missing variable may be the unique food sensitivities of different people. Particular sensitivities need to be identified, the offending foods eliminated, and the digestive system restored to its normal functioning. Allergists also stress the importance of proper digestion of foods. Even healthy food, if only partially digested, can be treated by the body as a toxin and stimulate an allergic response.

THE NO-NIGHTSHADE DIET

Early evidence that arthritis attacks can be triggered by specific foods was collected by retired horticulture professor Norman F. Childers, Ph.D., who developed the no-nightshade diet as an arthritis treatment in the 1970s. The food members of the nightshade family include potatoes, tomatoes, peppers, and eggplant. Peppers in the nightshade family include tabasco, cherry pepper, bell peppers, green peppers, chili peppers, red peppers, paprika—everything but black and white pepper, which are in a different family. Tobacco is also a nightshade, and so are the deadly and black nightshades used in making drugs, including belladonna, atropine, and scopolamine. The family of nightshades contains a chemical called solanine that seems to be toxic to everyone, although not everyone has a perceptible reaction to it. Robert Bingham, M.D., Medical Director at the Desert Arthritis and Medical Clinic in Desert Hot Springs, California, reports that approximately one-third of patients with rheumatoid arthritis are sensitive to the nightshades.[1]

In the folklore of foods, those in the nightshade family have been regarded with suspicion for centuries. Long ago, a society was formed in England for the specific purpose of discouraging the use of the potato as food. Tomatoes were also considered poisonous at one time; and eggplants were called the "apple of insanity," based on the belief that overconsumption would cause psychosis. Interestingly, solanine interferes with acetylcholine, a neurotransmitter needed for brain function. It also inhibits the action of cholinesterase, the enzyme that provides agility and flexibility in muscles.[2]

Dr. Childers discovered the relationship between the nightshades and joint pain by personal experience. He developed arthritis and diverticulitis in his fifties. All of his symptoms resolved when he quit drinking a hot spiced tomato drink of which he had been quite fond. One of his first clues to the link was his observation as a horticulturist that livestock wouldn't eat tomato plants if given a choice and developed arthritic joints if they did. Because his no-nightshade diet was promoted in the seventies, when conventional medicine still scoffed at the notion of a dietary component to the disease, his book *A Diet to Stop Arthritis* had little impact. Today, when dietary theories are again in vogue, it has been either ignored or discounted; but Dr. Childers did substantial research establishing the validity of his claims, conducting a nationwide survey involving thousands of volunteers. One reason the theory has been discounted may be the difficulty in testing it. Dr. Childers found that the nightshades had to be avoided for at least three months, and often for six to nine months, before results were seen. After that length of time, however, 72 percent of respondents reported experiencing improvement in their conditions. Enthusiasts reported that arthritis pain that had troubled them for years was gone in a matter of months. Gout also responded to the no-nightshade diet, and so did the locking of arthritic joints when in the "wrong" position.

Dr. Childers suspected that the percentage of people affected could actually be higher than that found in his study, since the nightshades are often hidden in the diet. Tomato sauce and hot pepper are ubiquitous in foods. Tomatoes are contained in ketchup, pizza, and tomato sauce. The jaded, overstimulated palate needs more and more hot pepper to give it a buzz. Paprika is used to color some packaged foods. Potato starch is used to thicken some yogurts. Potatoes are popular as french fries and potato chips, two forms that are particularly hazardous because solanine is increased in proportion to the number of surfaces exposed to light. At least one drug commonly prescribed for arthritics is also made from a nightshade. The drug is Lomotil, prescribed for digestive complaints; the nightshade derivative it contains is atropine.

Response to the no-nightshades diet is delayed by drugs, particularly cortisone or gold injections; so if you want to test the diet and you're taking those drugs, you should ask your doctor if you can reduce their intake for a while.[3]

THE ALLERGY FACTOR

Solanine is a toxin that inhibits the action of acetylcholine and cholinesterase in everyone. Allergic reactions, by contrast, are individualized responses to specific foods. That they can initiate, aggravate, or imitate arthritis is demonstrated by the relief afforded when offending foods have been removed from the diets of arthritics, and by the fresh attacks produced when these foods have been reintroduced.

The link between arthritis and allergic reactions was first pointed out in the 1950s by Theron G. Randolph, M.D., the founder of environmental medicine. He tested over 1,000 patients with commonly eaten foods and chemicals and found a significant connection to their arthritic complaints.

Connecticut allergist Marshall Mandell, M.D., has found that at least 80 percent of rheumatoid arthritics have an allergic condition in the joints and surrounding structures affected by the disease. Allergic reactions aggravate the swelling, redness, pain, and limitation of motion in the joints. Dr. Mandell postulates that there is also an allergy component in osteoarthritis and childhood arthritis. In a double-blind study of forty arthritis patients, he and a colleague found that arthritis symptoms were provoked by reactions to allergens in either the diet or the environment (house dust, molds, tobacco smoke, petrochemicals) for 86 percent of the patients studied. Most never suspected allergies as factors in their conditions.

In another study, about two-thirds of arthritics examined actually had an allergy-related disease. Arthritic symptoms could be relieved by the patients avoiding the particular dietary and environmental allergens.[4]

Dr. Mandell says an allergy component is likely if you have either a family or a personal history of allergies, or if your arthritis improves when fasting or gets worse after meals or on certain days or places. If you suspect allergies, keep a diary correlating possible exposures and symptoms and study it for clues.

HEREDITY OR BAD DIET?

Food allergies *may* be hereditary, but they may also be a response to bad diet and overeating of certain foods. Dr. Aesoph explains that nutritional deficiency caused by eating nutrient-deficient and enzyme-deficient processed foods paves the way for food allergies. These allergies, in turn, trigger an immune system attack on the tissue in the joints. When poor digestion only partially breaks food down, large food particles passing through the gut barrier are mistaken by the immune system for foreign invaders, setting off system-wide immune reactions. The foods that provoke these reactions are the allergenic foods specific to the individual. Usually, they are the foods eaten most often. Pesticides, fertilizers, and other chemicals on the food may spark reactions even if the food itself is healthy. Irradiation, pasteurization, and genetic engineering add fuel to the fire by structurally altering the molecules so the body has trouble recognizing them as food.[5]

HOME ALLERGY TESTING

Allergenic foods can be tracked down by clinical testing, but there are also ways to make this determination at home. These methods take patience and persistence and may not locate all allergies, since some reactions are delayed and hard to pin to specific foods; but if merely changing from a junk food to a natural whole-foods diet hasn't produced the desired results, they are worth a try.

One way to locate allergies without professional help is to go on an elimination diet in which suspect foods are omitted. The most frequent offenders are milk and milk products, wheat, yeast, corn, eggs, coffee, soy, potatoes, tomatoes, beef, pork, chicken, peanuts, oranges, chocolate, and sugar. Add suspect foods back in at the rate of one every second day. Keep careful notes of your dietary habits and symptoms and look for correlations, since an allergic response may not be immediate. It could take hours or even a couple of days. Before initiating the elimination diet, it is best to go on a short fast to clear the system.[6]

This protocol and its effectiveness were demonstrated in a randomized controlled Norwegian study discussed in chapter 8. Twenty-seven patients with RA were put on a seven- to ten-day modified fast consisting of herbal teas, garlic, vegetable broth, decoctions of potatoes and parsley, and juice extracts from carrots, beets, and celery. Energy intake during this "subtotal" fast was from 800 to 1260 calories per day. When the fast was completed, a new food with joint-aggravating potential was introduced into the diet every second day. If the suspect food exacerbated symptoms, it was eliminated from the diet for seven days. For the next three and one-half months the patients were not to eat meat, fish, eggs, dairy products, refined sugar, citrus fruits or foods containing gluten (a protein in most grains that aggravates many cases of arthritis). Also to be avoided were salt, strong spices, preservatives, alcoholic beverages, tea, and coffee. Cod liver oil was given as a vitamin D supplement. After three and one-half months the patients were allowed to reintroduce dairy and gluten products so long as symptoms were not exacerbated by them. The diet group showed a significant improvement in various objective and subjective indices of joint disease and pain after four weeks on this protocol, and the benefits were still present after one year.[7]

Dr. Carlton Fredericks suggests another easy home method for tracing possible allergens: take your pulse before and after eating suspect foods. First take it in the morning before getting up. Then eat just one suspect food a half hour later, then the same food an hour later. If the pulse has risen more than sixteen beats a minute, or to a total of more than eighty-four beats a minute, you are probably allergic to that food. The procedure is faster if done with full meals, but when your pulse races after a meal you still have to figure out which individual food did it.

Interestingly, the pulse test only works with foods you eat regularly. If you don't eat a food for a while, your body desensitizes itself to it. This phenomenon is the basis of the "rotation diet," in which you eat any one common offender no more often than once every four days. In the elapsed time, the body desensitizes to the food and isn't stressed when it is next consumed. For some people, however, a five- to eight-day rotation period is required for this to work; and for extremely sensitive people, no amount of time is enough. Likewise, no amount of time is enough to desensitize to the nightshades, which contain a toxic, not just allergenic, component. For nightshade toxicity, the no-nightshade diet remains the best alternative.[8]

NUTRITIONAL SUPPLEMENTS

Changing the diet from an unhealthy to a healthy one will help repair nutritional deficiencies, but it takes time. Nutritional supplements in pill form can speed the process. That therapeutic alternative is explored in Part Three.

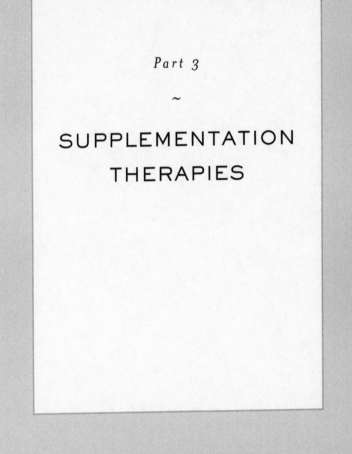

Part 3

~

SUPPLEMENTATION THERAPIES

Glucosamine and Chondroitin Sulfates: If Not a Cure, a Step in the Right Direction

> *Let us a little permit Nature to take her own way; she better understands her own affairs than we.*
>
> —MONTAIGNE,
> *Essays* (1580)

Nutritional supplements for relieving arthritis pain have suddenly become a craze. Leading the market is glucosamine, recommended by Jason Theodosakis, M.D., in his book *The Arthritis Cure.*[1] One hundred thousand copies of this 1997 bestseller were snatched up within three days of Dr. Theodosakis' appearance on the *Today* show. He maintains in his book that a combination of two nutritional supplements sold in health food stores, glucosamine and chondroitin sulfates, not only can relieve the pain of osteoarthritis but can regenerate deteriorating cartilage in the joints.

Sales of the supplements and the book were given a boost when *New York Times* health columnist Jane Brody reported using the supplements to treat her arthritic eleven-year-old spaniel. When the dog's condition improved, she tried the supplements for her own arthritic knees. After two months, she estimated her improvement at 30 percent.[2]

Osteoarthritis occurs, says Dr. Theodosakis, when the cartilage covering joints deteriorates faster than the body can replace it. Glucosamine and chondroitin sulfates are used continually in the joints to help produce healthy cartilage to cushion the ends of the bones and allow them to pivot smoothly. These two substances are found naturally in foods but in very small quantities. They pass through blood to the joints, where they stimulate the production of new cartilage cells and reduce the action of enzymes that harm cartilage. Both substances have been used for decades by veterinarians on ailing animal joints.

Both come as sulfates; they contain sulfur. Sulfur has been used for healing throughout history, and sulfur-rich mineral springs are perennially popular with arthritics. Sulfur is one of the raw materials necessary for making protein, connective tissue, and enzymes, making it essential for normal body function; yet it is typically overlooked in supplementing the body's mineral needs.

Glucosamine is a combination of sugar and an amino acid needed to build healthy cartilage. Chondroitin sulfate serves to draw fluid into the cartilage, protecting existing cartilage from premature breakdown. Taking these nutrients regularly in supplemental form helps bring cartilage production back into balance. Dr. Theodosakis cites fifteen studies done in Europe and Asia in which patients reported less pain when taking this nutrient combination. Critics contest whether it represents a true "cure," since claims that it reverses X ray evidence of joint damage have not been substantiated.[3] These same experts generally agree, however, that the touted nutrients relieve pain; and unlike aspirin and other NSAIDs (which also don't cure arthritis), the nutrients have no known side effects or adverse drug interactions. Dr. Theodosakis states that they have been given in dosages up to ten times those he recommends with no signs of toxicity.[4] The approach is thus clearly a step in the right direction. Unlike NSAIDs, it satisfies Hippocrates' injunction to "First do no harm."

GLUCOSAMINE RESEARCH

The European and Asian clinical trials generally showed that patients with mild to moderate arthritis get relief from glucosamine. Symptomatic relief was reported in 50 to 80 percent of the treatment groups as compared to 20 to 30 percent of the placebo groups. These effects weren't permanent, but they could last for several months after therapy. Reported side effects were mild and mostly gastrointestinal.[5]

In several double-blind European studies comparing glucosamine to arthritis drugs such as ibuprofen, glucosamine provided pain relief equivalent to the drugs. Although it took longer to work—perhaps several weeks—the reason the drugs worked more quickly was that they were suppressing a natural function, leading directly to their potentially serious side effects.[6] Glucosamine is without adverse effects because it supports rather than counteracts the body's own efforts at healing.

A double-blind study from the People's Republic of China reported in 1998 found that glucosamine sulfate actually worked better than NSAIDs. The subjects, 178 Chinese patients suffering from osteoarthritis of the knee, were randomly assigned to two groups. One group was treated for four weeks with 1,500 mg daily of glucosamine sulfate. The other group was treated with 1,200 mg daily of ibuprofen. Glucosamine was found to be both better tolerated and more effective in reducing symptoms than the popular drug.[7]

A double-blind study done in Spain involved 329 people divided into four groups. For three months, one group was given the standard antiarthritis drug piroxicam (Feldene), a second was given glucosamine, a third received both treatments, and a fourth received only a placebo (an inert preparation). Piroxicam and glucosamine proved equally effective at reducing symptoms during the treatment period; and the combination treatment (piroxicam plus glucosamine) did not produce significantly better results than either treatment taken alone. After treatment was stopped, the patients were followed for an additional two months. The benefits of piroxicam rapidly disappeared, but the benefits of glucosamine lasted for the full two months.[8]

Unfortunately, the FDA does not recognize the validity of foreign studies; and American studies are sparse. *The Medical Letter on Drugs and Therapeutics,* a newsletter for doctors, therefore drew up its own panel of experts to review the acceptable evidence. The experts acknowledged that in laboratory tests, glucosamine had been found to stimulate the synthesis of cartilage; and that the incidence of side effects was very low. But human trials, said the *Letter,* were short-term. As of the date of that report (1997), whether glucosamine had lasting benefits remained inconclusive.[9]

New studies are coming out all the time, however, and most demonstrate significant pain relief. They show that glucosamine not only works as well as NSAIDs but that reductions in pain and swelling and improvements in mobility can continue for weeks after treatment stops, suggesting it does more than simply suppress symptoms. Progressive joint damage also seems to be delayed, slowing the course of the disease.[10] In a three-year, double-blind, placebo-controlled American study of 212 patients reported in 1999, the patients given glucosamine showed improvement in pain and mobility over the course of the study, while those given a placebo worsened steadily during the same period. X rays also showed that glucosamine treatment prevented progressive damage to the knee joint.[11] In a study reported in *The Lancet* on January 27, 2001, 70 patients with arthritis of the knee were given glucosamine, while a similar number took a placebo for three years. Most had mild arthritis not requiring pain medication. In the placebo group, the space between the bones in the knee joint got smaller (objective evidence that arthritis had progressed), while in the glucosamine group it did not. Compared to drugs, which can actually speed the disease process, glucosamine thus appears to represent a revolutionary breakthrough in the treatment of arthritis.[12]

Not all studies, however, have been positive. A two-month, double-blind, placebo-controlled trial of 98 people with osteoarthritis of the knee reported in 2000 found no benefit from treatment with glucosamine. The researchers suggested the relatively advanced osteoarthritis found in these patients was responsible for the negative results. Negative results were also reported in a 1999 double-blind, placebo-controlled trial of glucosamine hydrochloride.[13]

No significant side effects have been reported in any of the glucosamine studies, suggesting it is quite safe for people of all ages. Recent case reports and animal studies have raised concerns, however, that glucosamine could be harmful for people with diabetes, since it can raise blood sugar levels and may increase the risk of long-term diabetic side effects such as cataracts. There is also a potential sensitivity problem for people with allergies to shrimp, lobster and crab, from which glucosamine supplements are derived.[14]

CHONDROITIN SULFATE STUDIES

The demonstrated benefits of chondroitin sulfate have been mainly from its injectable form. Chondroitin sulfate was thought to be poorly absorbed from the digestive tract, raising the question whether supplementing it along with glucosamine in capsule form would do any good. But in 1998, a Swiss study reported positive results with the supplements. Joint pain was significantly reduced in 42 patients with osteoarthritis of the knee after taking chondroitin sulfate orally for three months as compared to a placebo group. After they took it for six months, mobility was also significantly increased.[15]

Still to be answered is whether the mechanism of action of chondroitin sulfate differs from that of glucosamine, and whether using the two in combination is more effective than using either alone. Preliminary information from one 1999 animal study suggests that the mixture may be superior to either treatment alone.[16]

SOURCES AND DOSES

Glucosamine is available not only as glucosamine sulfate but as glucosamine hydrochloride and N-acetyl-glucosamine (NAG), as well as in shark cartilage and cow cartilage. All are sold as tablets or capsules. Which works best is disputed, but glucosamine sulfate is the likely winner, since it is better absorbed and provides bioavailable sulfur, a mineral that helps provide the protein links necessary for cartilage repair.[17]

Dr. Theodosakis suggests starting with 1,000 mg of glucosamine and 800 mg of chondroitin sulfate daily if you weigh less than 120 pounds; 1,500 mg and 1,200 mg, respectively, if you weigh 120 to 200 pounds; or 2,000 mg and 1,600 mg, respectively, if you weigh more than 200 pounds. As pain decreases, gradually decrease the dose. Then be patient. Results can take weeks to develop. Allow eight weeks before abandoning the endeavor.

Another source of cartilage that is cheap and readily available is plain gelatin powder, mixed in juice and drunk uncooked. To blend it, fill a blender half full with any kind of juice, then "pulse" one cup of plain gelatin into it, a bit at a time. Return this mixture to a half-gallon container, fill the container to the top with juice, stir, then put it in the refrigerator overnight. Drink one-half cup of this juice mixture twice a day.

EXPLAINING VARIABLE RESULTS

In my own case, when I first tried a course of glucosamine sulfate, I felt no discernible improvement in my arthritic hip. I believe, however, that this was because my pain was from toxic accumulation in the joint. Rebuilding cartilage won't eliminate these toxins. After I removed those blocks to healing through fasting, a niacin flush, homeopathic chelation remedies (discussed in chapter 27), and the repair of an infected molar tooth (discussed in chapter 24), my hip no longer bothered me. The problem at that time was my neck, which had begun to hurt from intensive work bending over a laptop computer. A chiropractor reported that his manual examination suggested arthritis was developing there. I tried another course of a high-quality glucosamine and chondroitin sulfate combination and on that occasion found that, at the maximum recommended dose of 2,000 mg per day, it eased my neck pain within eight hours of taking it.

The difference may have been in the tuned-up ability of my body to use these supplemental nutrients. Discrepancies in the results of studies on the effectiveness of glucosamine and other natural remedies could have similar explanations. Supplying missing nutrients is only part of the equation. Joint-irritating toxins and blockages to healing must also be removed. Another variable could be the quality of the supplements used. Some supplements have been found to contain substantially less of the active ingredients than claimed on their labels.

QUALITY AND QUANTITY CONTROL

This brings up a general caution relevant to all the nutritional supplements discussed in this section. Vitamin and mineral supplements are one category of product in which you usually get what you pay for. Supplements should be of high quality and in bioavailable form. Capsules, which contain powder, are easier to digest than tablets. While good nutritional supplements can be quite effective, overdosing on handfuls of cheap, hard-to-digest tablets may make arthritis worse, since they are difficult for people with weak digestions to metabolize. Calcium supplements are particular hazards. Women who take handfuls of hard calcium tablets or Tums thinking they are preventing osteoporosis can actually be contributing to joint disease, because calcium that is not metabolized settles out in the joints and tissues.

An excellent database on nutritional supplements called *The Natural Pharmacy* is available on the Internet at www.TNP.com. Mail-order sources of good high-quality nutritional supplements include Pacific Research Laboratories in Torrance, California (telephone 800-325-7734), and the Golden Cabinet in Sag Harbor, New York (telephone 631-725-5720).

FIFTEEN

While You Heal: Safer Pain Relief with DMSO and MSM

[DMSO] has fallen out of the limelight and out of the main-stream of medical discourse, leading some to believe that it was discredited. The truth is more complicated . . .

—MAYA MUIR,
"DMSO" (1997)[1]

While glucosamine sulfate and other nutritional supplements take days or weeks to work, this isn't true for DMSO (dimethyl sulfoxide). Like aspirin and other NSAIDs, DMSO can relieve pain immediately. Unlike those drugs, it does not work by suppressing prostaglandin synthesis or have dangerous side effects. It reduces pain by addressing the cause, attack by free radicals on the joints. DMSO works by binding with them, thus counteracting free radical insults to the joints.

DMSO is classified as a drug and is controversial, but I feel compelled to write on it because it worked so well for me. When I needed a "quick fix" for joint pain on a sleepless night or a long plane ride, it gave fast relief without side effects. The form I like is a rose-scented cream in an aloe vera base, obtainable from DMSO Marketing Inc., telephone (800) 367-6935.

HISTORY AND VICISSITUDES

DMSO has been the subject of some 11,000 articles internationally on its medical and clinical uses, making it one of the most studied pharmaceutical agents of our time. Drug companies were at one time hotly competing for it. The reasons it hasn't yet passed the FDA as an arthritis treatment are bound up with politics, economics, and the unmistakable odor of its liquid form.

The only established side effect of liquid DMSO is its pronounced garlic odor, an odd characteristic that precludes the kind of double-blind studies required for FDA approval, since recipients always know they are getting the drug. But animals, which aren't subject to the placebo effect, respond very well to DMSO, making it another popular veterinary remedy for joint problems; and on humans with arthritis, DMSO has an established success record in other countries. It is widely available in the United States and is inexpensive.[2] It is also available in a cream form, which produces no unpleasant odor that I can detect; but the impetus for testing DMSO clinically as an arthritis cure has now passed, so studies proving the effectiveness of this cream are not likely to be forthcoming in the near future.

Originally synthesized by a Russian chemist in the late nineteenth century, DMSO was the first nonsteroidal anti-inflammatory to be discovered after aspirin. A natural product made from the lignin that binds wood fiber together in trees, DMSO is used commercially as a paint thinner, solvent, and additive to chemical products. Its medical potential was discovered when Crown Zellerbach Paper Company asked Robert Herschler, the company's chemist in charge of research, to find another profitable use for it. Dr. Herschler observed that DMSO moved through the tissues of plants and trees and carried other materials with it. The same proved to be true in animals, making it of interest for carrying medicines into the body through the skin.

Dr. Herschler discovered DMSO's therapeutic properties by accident, when he used it on a blister from a chemical burn. The blister immediately disappeared, along with the pain of the burn. In the 1950s he met Stanley Jacob, a surgeon whose interest in DMSO stemmed from his work in kidney transplant technology. DMSO was a chemical compound that permitted the freezing of red blood cells in a way that retained their viability for transplantation. Together, these two scientists began exploring DMSO's medical possibilities.

DMSO was found to have strong pain-reducing and anti-inflammatory properties. Applied topically, it enters the bloodstream and seeks out water like a magnet. It goes to swollen areas; latches onto the blood, lymph fluid, or pus collected there; and moves them into the bloodstream. When the liquid leaves, the swelling subsides and so does the pain. DMSO also increases the effectiveness of the body's own anti-inflammatory hormone cortisol (the natural form of cortisone).

Patients being treated by Dr. Jacob were soon reporting on the remarkable ability of DMSO to relieve pain, particularly from various forms of arthritis. It was hailed as the latest wonder drug. Drug companies sought it for use in transporting their patented drugs into the body through the skin, thereby bypassing the digestive tract, where adverse reactions often occur.

But there were impediments to DMSO's development. One was that it was already on the market, and no company could acquire an exclusive patent for its medical use. As noted earlier, without a patent, manufacturers cannot make enough money from the product to cover the more than $100 million now required to get a single drug or device past the FDA. And since DMSO was already available for industrial use as a solvent, patients could dose themselves. When word got out about its remarkable effects on various intractable conditions, people started doing just that, leading to uncontrolled experimentation and an eventual souring of the medical community on it.

There was an initial flurry of interest in DMSO in the sixties, when six pharmaceutical companies began clinical studies. Then in 1965, a woman in Ireland died of an allergic reaction after taking DMSO along with several other drugs. The exact cause of death was never determined, but DMSO got the blame. Two months later, the FDA closed down clinical trials in the United States, citing the woman's death and changes in the eyes of certain laboratory animals that had been given doses of the drug many times higher than would be given to humans. After twenty years of research involving hundreds of laboratory and human studies, no further deaths have been reported, and no changes in the eyes of humans have been documented. The FDA has nevertheless refused seven applications to conduct clinical studies. Dr. Jacob suggests that the FDA, influenced by drug interests, actually "blackballed" the product, actively trying to kill interest in something that would compete with drugs already on the market or in development.[3]

FOREIGN STUDIES

The FDA has approved the prescriptive use of DMSO only for interstitial cystitis (inflammation of the bladder). However, research in other countries has clearly established its therapeutic benefits for many other conditions including arthritis. Here are some recent arthritis studies:

In a German study, patients with acute tendon pain were randomized to receive either a topical DMSO gel or a placebo. After fourteen days, 44 percent of the DMSO recipients were pain free, compared to only 9 percent of those on placebo.

DMSO was well tolerated and produced no "severe undesired events." The researchers concluded that DMSO is suitable for topical use, producing clinically relevant results with little risk to the patient.[4]

In a second double-blind German study involving 112 patients with arthritic knees, DMSO gel was found to have a "clinically relevant analgesic effect" on pain during everyday activities as compared to a placebo.[5]

In a double-blind Russian study on patients with rheumatoid arthritis, objective favorable effects, including an increase in hand strength, were documented after topical application of DMSO.[6]

In a second Russian study, DMSO was found to have greater therapeutic effects than the conventional drug colchicine on the kidney symptoms of patients with rheumatoid arthritis.[7]

In a Russian study involving mice, DMSO lessened the destructive changes in the joints and inhibited the development of spontaneous chronic arthritis.[8]

In an Australian study, arthritis was induced in rats by injecting tuberculosis bacteria. Clinical evidence of arthritis was significantly reduced by treatment with DMSO over a two-week period.[9]

In an Italian study, patients with rheumatoid arthritis experienced a decrease in inflammatory activity and relief of symptoms after using oral DMSO. No serious side effects occurred except for an unpleasant breath odor.[10]

In another study, DMSO stimulated healing and protected against the complications of hemorrhage from NSAIDs in patients with either osteoarthritis or rheumatoid arthritis. Fifty-eight of these patients were given 500 mg of DMSO orally four times daily. Endoscopic examination showed that only 7 percent of them had erosive gastritis (stomach erosions), compared to 50 percent of the 59 patients in the control group.[11]

PRECAUTIONS

One of DMSO's unique properties is that it carries other molecules with it into the cells. This property can be not only a boon but a hazard, since DMSO can carry pesticides and other pollutants along with it. For that reason, users should take care to have quite clean skin at the application site. Only pure DMSO should be used, not the less refined commercial versions used in industry. Drs. Herschler and Jacob recommend not using DMSO at strengths greater than 70 percent dilution, and not using it every day. Five days out of seven are good.[12]

MSM

MSM (methyl sulphonyl methane or $DMSO_2$) is DMSO's major metabolite and breakdown product. It was developed as a therapeutic remedy specifically to overcome the drawback of the objectionable garlic odor of DMSO. The tradeoff is that the relief MSM affords is not as immediate as for DMSO. Like glucosamine sulfate, MSM is a nontoxic organic sulfur compound that aids the repair of damaged tissue and takes days or weeks to work. Unlike glucosamine, MSM has not been extensively studied. But according to Dr. Jacob, the physician who first recommended it to patients nearly twenty years ago, it has proven in his clinical practice to be more effective in reducing the pain and inflammation of arthritis than glucosamine.[13] Like DMSO and glucosamine, MSM is a popular veterinary product that has been around for decades, with a proven track record for relieving joint stiffness in dogs and horses.

Its use on human patients goes back to when Dr. Jacob started recommending it for people attending his DMSO Clinic at the Oregon Health Sciences University in Portland. People typically went to the Portland clinic only as a last resort after conventional treatments had been tried and failed. It was on these seriously ill people that Dr. Jacob first observed MSM's remarkable health benefits. He had observed that while DMSO, the parent compound, was highly effective, many people using it for chronic conditions stopped taking it because of its objectionable odor. MSM proved to have most of the benefits of DMSO without the odor. Benefits included reduction of inflammation, inhibition of pain impulses along the nerve fibers, an increase in blood supply, reduction in muscle spasm, softening of scar tissue, relief from allergies, an increase in energy, relief of constipation, softer skin, thicker hair, and stronger nails.

Cases cited by Dr. Jacob and his co-authors include a woman with arthritis in the knees, whose pain was substantially reduced after taking MSM for two to three months; a mail carrier with arthritic knees, whose pain was entirely eliminated and who avoided surgery by taking MSM; a woman who suffered from fibromyalgia for five years, which was largely relieved after three weeks on MSM; a severe case of TMJ (temporomandibular joint disorder or pain in the jaw joint) that largely cleared up, although the process took a number of months; and a disabling case of whiplash, which was completely resolved in two months.[14]

Like glucosamine, MSM doesn't permanently cure arthritis. If you stop taking it, your pain will probably come back. But again this is also true for the widely prescribed NSAIDs; and unlike those drugs, MSM has no unwanted side effects. It takes longer to act than NSAIDs, but this is because it is a nutrient. Rather than masking pain by suppressing a natural body function, MSM addresses the cause. In some cases, it can produce results in a matter of days, easing pain and increasing energy and an overall sense of well-being. In tough cases, however, the process may take months, so you are advised not to give up if you haven't gotten results after a short-term trial.

Like DMSO, MSM is FDA-approved in the United States for use only in treating interstitial cystitis. It is used in other countries in the treatment of arthritis, however, as well as for muscle and skeletal problems, athletic injuries, and other ailments. It is also a valuable aid in offsetting the toxic effects of chronic mercury exposure. Mercury has a great affinity for the sulfur molecule.[15]

MSM is available in health food stores without a prescription and is inexpensive. It comes as capsules, in crystal form (to be mixed with juice), and as creams, lotions, or gels for topical application. The recommended dose for general purposes is around two grams (2,000 mg) daily, although many patients have needed three or four grams or more daily to experience therapeutic effects, and athletes have taken five or more grams before and after workouts to increase stamina and reduce muscle soreness. A level kitchen teaspoon holds about one gram of MSM crystals.[16] MSM is also found in most natural unprocessed foods; but it is lost when fresh food is cooked, processed, or stored. The richest natural source of MSM is mother's milk.[17]

SIXTEEN

Herbal Arthritis Remedies

O! mickle is the powerful grace that lies
In herbs, plants, stones, and their true qualities.

—SHAKESPEARE,
Romeo and Juliet

Other safe and inexpensive derivatives from the plant world are natural analgesics and anti-inflammatories that can afford relief for arthritis sufferers.

CAPSAICIN

One natural option that is supported by research and is widely available in drugstores is topical capsaicin, a cream sold over the counter under several names, including Zostrix, ToppSation, and Capsaicin. Topical capsaicin is not an arthritis "cure" but is a good alternative to drugs for immediate short-term relief, since unlike NSAIDs, it is without side effects except for a biting sensation like the sting of hot pepper on the tongue. Despite this warmth or burning feeling on the skin, it does not raise skin temperature or cause blistering. The "picante" sensation comes from its active ingredient, which is actually derived from red chili peppers. Ironically, these nightshades, which can provoke a toxic reaction if eaten, can relieve pain when applied to the skin. The proposed mechanism is that capsaicin reduces something called "substance P," a neuropeptide that carries pain signals. With less substance P in your tissues, fewer nerve impulses are sent to the spinal cord, so you feel less pain.

James Duke, Ph.D., a retired Department of Agriculture botanist, says using hot sauce or hot peppers directly on the skin is just as effective as using the drugstore capsaicin products. Using the natural sauce also avoids any of the potentially objectionable chemicals added to commercial creams. Dr. Duke's recipe involves saturating gauze or a cotton ball with hot sauce and applying it to painful joints; or mixing one-half teaspoon chopped hot pepper (chopped while wearing gloves) with a cup of warm vegetable oil, then rubbing this mixture into ailing joints.[1]

CAPSAICIN STUDIES

Studies have demonstrated capsaicin's effectiveness in relieving the pain of both osteoarthritis and rheumatoid arthritis. In one well-designed study, the participants applied either capsaicin cream or a placebo cream four times daily to the front, back, and sides of the knee. All had suffered moderate to very severe knee pain. Pain relief for the capsaicin users was significantly greater than for those using the placebo. A burning sensation was noted by nearly half the capsaicin users, but this effect either decreased or disappeared with repeated use. The dosage used (0.025 percent) was similar to that in over-the-counter products.[2] In another study, from the Medical College of Wisconsin, a 0.075 percent capsaicin cream applied four times daily produced good results.

Vanderbilt University researchers writing in *The Annals of Internal Medicine* in 1994 studied several nonmedical treatments for osteoarthritis, including diathermy (deep heat), laser therapy, TENS (transcutaneous nerve stimulation) therapy, and topical capsaicin. Although diathermy did not seem to help, the other treatments, including topical capsaicin, did. The researchers observed that the considerable risks associated with the use of nonsteroidal anti-inflammatory drugs in older populations are now being recognized, making these natural alternatives attractive options for physicians. Yet medical trials of promising alternative therapies are scarce. The reason, they suggested, is that studies of nonmedical therapies usually have no clear financial sponsor.[3]

CAUTIONS

Users are warned to apply topical capsaicin sparingly and to keep it away from the eyes, other delicate areas, and sores or open cuts. They are also advised not to count on it working overnight. Regular applications are the key to pain relief.

In my own case, a drugstore capsaicin cream did work overnight, but I prefer DMSO cream because it lacks the burning sensation of capsaicin. However, I would use either before NSAIDs.

OTHER HERBAL OPTIONS

Other herbs also act as natural analgesics and anti-inflammatories. One with potent anti-inflammatory and antioxidant properties that have been verified by clinical studies is ginger. Ginger also works like capsaicin or cayenne by cutting substance P levels. For RA, a daily oral dose of two to four grams of dry powdered ginger is suggested, or one-half inch of sliced fresh ginger root.

Another herb with particularly strong anti-inflammatory

properties is curcumin, a component of turmeric, the yellow ingredient in curry powder. Curcumin has been shown to be as effective as cortisone in suppressing inflammation, without its side effects. Turmeric can be sprinkled on food, used in curried dishes, or taken as supplements available in health food stores. It may also be mixed with lime juice and used as a poultice to relieve aching joints.[4]

Boswellia is a third herb used in the treatment of arthritis. In one study of 175 patients with RA, 97 percent of them achieved "fair to excellent" results using boswellic extracts; and no side effects were reported. The standard dosage is 400 mg three times daily.

Devil's claw, an herb native to Africa, has been shown in animal studies to have anti-inflammatory and analgesic effects equivalent to the powerful NSAID phenylbutazone. The recommended daily dose is one to two grams taken as dried powdered root or made into a cup of tea.

An extract of yucca was also shown to be of benefit on RA in a double-blind clinical trial. The recommended dose is two to four grams taken as powdered yucca leaf or as a tea.

Chinese thoroughwax contains steroid-like compounds with significant anti-inflammatory action. It is sometimes recommended for patients on steroid drugs, to help protect the adrenal gland.[5]

The herb feverfew has been shown to be more effective at inhibiting inflammation and fever than aspirin. The herbal form of aspirin is willow bark. Used by Chinese physicians 2,500 years ago, it contains salicin, nearly the same pain reliever found in aspirin. Another herbal "aspirin" is meadowsweet tea. These herbs have been reported to relieve pain as effectively as aspirin at much lower risk.[6]

Herbal options good for gout include devil's claw, burdock tea or capsules, and celery seed capsules or tea. Better yet is

SEVENTEEN

Enzymes, Digestive Aids, and Dietary Habits

No mineral, vitamin or hormone can do any work without enzymes. The body may have the raw building materials, but without the workers, it cannot begin.

—EDWARD HOWELL, M.D.[1]

Other supplements found to be highly effective for arthritis relief are digestive and pancreatic enzymes. Supplemental enzymes have been shown to reduce inflammation and joint pain not only in osteoarthritis but in the more intractable rheumatoid arthritis, and they do it without the daunting side effects of conventional drugs.

Research traces the underlying problem to the modern diet. Cooking, microwaving, and processing destroy enzymes found naturally in foods. As a result, food gets to the colon undigested, leaving toxic residues that must be detoxified by the liver. When the liver becomes overloaded, toxins enter the blood, where they can evoke an aggressive autoimmune response and the production of circulating immune complexes. (See chapter 5.) Deteriorating joints also produce corrosive proteins leading to the production of immune complexes, which lodge in the joints and cause irritation. The problem can affect all forms of cherry juice, a remarkably effective treatment for gout. Some component of cherries stops uric acid crystals from forming. For prevention, either drink the juice or eat ten to fifteen cherries daily.[7]

Combination products are available that allow you to take a range of herbs and other nutrients that promote joint health in one tablet. One that I like is called Arth-X Plus and contains yucca, devil's claw, burdock root, chaparral, Mexican sarsaparilla root, capsicum, and hydrangea, along with glucosamine sulfate and a long list of other nutrients. It is made by Trace Minerals in Roy, Utah, and is available by mail order from the Golden Cabinet, telephone 631-725-5720.

A natural topical "quick fix" that has worked well for me is oil of citronella, an essential oil from Indonesia used in traditional Chinese medicine for relief of arthritic and rheumatic pain. It can be ordered off the Internet at *www.aromamarket.com*.

arthritis but is magnified in people with RA, who tend to be deficient in digestive enzymes (secreted by the pancreas) and in hydrochloric acid (secreted in the stomach). When proteins are not broken down properly by the pancreatic enzymes specific for their digestion, large molecules are left that are treated by the body as foreign, evoking an autoimmune response.[2]

Supplemental enzymes derived from plants can aid digestion in the stomach, and supplemental enzymes derived from the pancreases of animals can aid digestion in the intestines. Pancreatic enzyme formulations help by splitting the corrosive protein products that lead to joint inflammation into smaller chains of amino acids, which can then be eliminated from the system. These pancreatic preparations have been shown to be at least as effective as NSAIDs and other anti-inflammatory drugs in treating a variety of conditions including arthritis, but their side effects are very low. The preparations that have been extensively studied have usually involved combinations of the enzymes bromelain and trypsin.[3]

Caution: Supplemental enzymes are not recommended for people with bleeding disorders, inflammation of the intestines, reflux, or ulcers.

PANCREATIC ENZYMES

Although a number of pancreatic enzyme formulations are on the market, the one that has been most thoroughly studied is a bestselling German product called Wobenzym developed in the 1960s. Wobenzym tablets are pancreatic enzymes that are enteric coated to prevent digestion in the stomach, ensuring that they are liberated in the small intestine, where they share the workload of the body's own pancreatic enzymes. Wobenzym contains the enzymes trypsin, chymotrypsin, bromelain, papain, and pancreatin, with a small amount of the bioflavanoid rutin.

Among other studies, one published in the German medical journal *Natur- und Ganzheitsmedizin* in 1988 found that Wobenzym produced benefits for RA patients similar to those of gold therapy, without its toxic side effects.

Another study was reported in 1996 at the Second Russian Symposium on Oral Enzyme Therapy in St. Petersburg. The Russian researchers tested Wobenzym on seventy-eight patients with severe, crippling RA who were using other drugs for their disease. All of the patients showed a decrease in circulating immune complex concentrations (averaging between 28 and 42 percent) and decreases in rheumatoid factors. Twenty percent of the patients reduced their NSAID doses by 50 to 75 percent. One patient stopped taking the powerful but highly toxic drug methotrexate and experienced a clinical remission of the disease. Morning stiffness scores also improved. More than half the patients using Wobenzym rated their treatments as good, while only about a third of the patients using only medical drugs gave them this rating.

At the same conference, researchers presented findings on Wobenzym and juvenile arthritis. In the study, from the Paediatric Clinic of the Institute of Rheumatology of the Russian Academy of Medical Science, ten children with the disease were given five tablets of Wobenzym three times a day. They could also receive treatment with one NSAID in addition to Wobenzym. The number of actively inflamed joints was reduced from 44 to 15 by the second month, with general effectiveness being experienced after four to five months of treatment.[4]

The problem with most nutritional supplements is that they work so slowly that it is hard to tell which ones have helped. In my case, this was not true for Wobenzym tablets, which had a quite noticeable therapeutic effect within a few days. Wobenzym tablets are manufactured by MUCOS Pharma GmbH and are available by mail order from Naturally Vitamins in Scottsdale, Arizona, telephone 800-899-4499. They should be taken on an empty stomach, not less than forty-five minutes before or two hours after meals.

SUPPLEMENTS TO AID DIGESTION IN THE STOMACH

To aid digestion in the stomach, plant enzyme and hydrochloric acid tablets or capsules may be taken with meals. Plant enzymes are also obtainable from live, raw, unprocessed fruits and vegetables in the diet. Bromelain may be obtained from fresh pineapple, from which it is derived. Papain's natural source is fresh unripe papaya.

OTHER AIDS TO DIGESTION

Good digestion is not merely a matter of taking digestive aids. Foods must also be eaten at the right time and in the right combination. Even healthy food can do the body harm if overindulged in or taken in wrong combinations. Small frequent meals are easier to digest than fewer large ones. As Shakespeare noted, digestion should wait on appetite. We tend to eat as an escape or social outlet or according to a schedule, without listening to our stomachs. One of the benefits of fasting is that it helps you get in tune with your body and teaches you that you can skip a meal and actually feel the better for it.

Naturopathic writer Herbert M. Shelton stressed the importance of proper food combining, a theory based on the premise that different foods require different digestive enzymes. Foods such as fruits that may take only a few minutes to digest if eaten alone will be trapped and putrefy in the stomach if combined with foods taking many hours to digest. The basic rules are to avoid combining protein and starch in the same meal and to eat fruit alone. The theory was revived in the 1990s in several bestselling books, including *Fit for Life, The New Beverly Hills Diet,* and *Suzanne Somers' Eat Great, Lose Weight.*[5] The scientific basis of the theory has been disputed, but many people are convinced by personal experience that it works.

My own usual regimen is fruit salad with a good natural yogurt for breakfast, grains and greens for lunch, and a protein meal for dinner. If desserts or bad food combinations such as meats with carbohydrates must be eaten, dinner is considered the best time to do it, because digestion is stronger then. Animals in nature eat in quantity at sundown.

THE OFTEN OVERLOOKED IMPORTANCE OF DRINKING WATER

Water dilutes the digestive juices and should not be taken in quantity with meals, particularly by people with poor digestion. But drinking large quantities of water is still important. Fereydoon Batmanghelidj, M.D., in his book *Your Body's Many Cries for Water,* links the major chronic epidemics of modern life, including arthritis, to water dehydration. He reports cases in which arthritis and other chronic diseases were relieved simply by drinking sufficient amounts of water.

The body parts that suffer most from water dehydration, says Dr. Batmanghelidj, are those without direct vascular circulation, especially the joint cartilages in the fingers, knees, and vertebrae. Drinking sufficient water can cause pains to disappear and allow the joint to begin to repair itself. Other conditions that have been reversed include high blood pressure, low back pain, asthma, allergies, and ulcers. The regimen is also a good way to lose weight.

Our mistake, says Dr. Batmanghelidj, is in thinking we have satisfied our need for water by satisfying our thirst with other beverages. We need half our body's weight in ounces of water per day. A 128-pound woman, for example, would need 64 ounces or eight glasses of water. That means plain water (filtered or bottled)—not coffee, tea, alcohol, juices, soft drinks, or other manufactured beverages, which do contain water but also contain dehydrating agents. These cause the body to lose not only the water in which they are dissolved but additional water from the body's reserves.

Dr. Batmanghelidj advises waiting one-half hour before meals and two and one-half hours after meals for your heavy water doses, to avoid diluting your digestive juices; and adding one-half teaspoon of salt to your diet daily for every ten glasses of water added. Increase your water intake gradually to make sure your kidneys are functioning properly. Urine output should increase proportionately with water intake.

In recommending an *increased* salt intake, Dr. Batmanghelidj differs with modern medical opinion but agrees with ancient wisdom. He notes that Pliny the Elder called salt "foremost among human remedies." Salt is stored in the bones as crystals and is necessary to make them hard. The current emphasis on salt-free diets, Dr. Batmanghelidj asserts, could be contributing to osteoporosis.[6]

Other authorities attribute the high blood pressure resulting in some people when they increase their salt intakes not to salt itself but to the very high temperatures used in processing table salt, which transforms it into an unusable compound that the body regards as a foreign toxin. This problem can be avoided by using unheated sea salt.

EIGHTEEN

Cod Liver Oil, Vitamin D, Solar Therapy, and Cetyl Myristoleate

Truly the light is sweet, and a pleasant thing it is for the eyes to behold the sun.

—ECCLESIASTES 11:7

A daily dose of cod liver oil was once a favorite folk remedy for arthritic joints. When the steroids became popular, cod liver oil was essentially forgotten, but medical research has now confirmed its usefulness. Cod liver oil provides omega-3 fatty acids, which reduce inflammation; is an excellent source of vitamin A; and is the best natural food source of vitamin D. Vitamin D is particularly important for the joints because it aids the absorption of calcium, making calcium available for deposit in the bones. Increasing vitamin D intake to appropriate levels has been shown to cause calcium absorption to triple. If vitamin D is deficient, calcium is not metabolized but settles in the tissues and between the joints, creating aches and pains.

In a study conducted at the Brusch Medical Center in Cambridge, Massachusetts, ninety-eight people with various forms of arthritis (osteo-, rheumatoid, and gout) were instructed to take cod liver oil in the morning on an empty stomach. Ninety-three percent showed major improvement and 90 percent showed favorable changes in blood chemistry. A marked reduction in pain and an increase in energy and well-being were experienced in as little as two weeks, and blood sedimentation rates (measuring the severity of inflammation) dropped dramatically and consistently over a period of two to five months.[1]

A study showing that osteoarthritis may respond to a component of vitamin D was published in the September 1, 1996, issue of the *Annals of Internal Medicine*. The researchers looked at the records of people in the Framingham Heart Study with X-ray evidence of osteoarthritis in the knees. People least likely to have further degeneration later in life were found to be those with diets and blood levels high in vitamin D. Although the recommended daily allowance of vitamin D is only 200 IU, the best results occurred among people taking between two and eight times that amount. The researchers suggested that the vitamin's contribution is linked to its beneficial effects on the surrounding bone.[2]

Natural sources of vitamin D are preferred. Besides being in fish oil, vitamin D is available in egg yolk, milk, and butter (due to fortification). The vitamin D produced commercially, called vitamin D_2 (ergocalciferol), isn't the same as the vitamin D manufactured by the body (vitamin D_3). Vitamin D_3 isn't a true vitamin but is a hormone (cholecalciferol) produced in response to ultraviolet radiation. Taking vitamin D_2 orally is not only largely ineffective and unnatural but potentially dangerous in high doses. Cod liver oil remains the best food source of the biologically active form of vitamin D.[3]

Our most ubiquitous and available source, however, is still the sun. Vitamin D is produced in the body only after sunlight striking the skin initiates a series of reactions there.[4]

SUNLIGHT AS AN ARTHRITIS THERAPY

Studies show that blood levels of vitamin D are only weakly correlated with dietary intake. A much stronger correlation has been shown with exposure to sunlight. The evidence for this association is particularly compelling because it comes from England, where the sun rarely shines. British studies show that the sun is the principal source of vitamin D even when it isn't shining. A summer holiday at the beach, even for the British, affords better protection against vitamin D deficiency in the winter than vitamin D supplements. Residents of an old people's home who could spend some time in the garden were found to have normal vitamin D levels, while those confined indoors did not.[5]

Ultraviolet (UV) light from the sun is good for the joints and bones because it aids calcium absorption into the skeleton. When calcium is ingested but isn't absorbed into the bones, extraskeletal calcium can wind up getting deposited in the tissues and joints and along the walls of the arteries, contributing to arteriosclerosis (hardening of the arteries). Phototherapy pioneer John Ott showed that laboratory animals raised under artificial lighting developed excessive calcium deposits in their hearts, lost their hair, and developed large, fast-growing tumors.[6]

A study of elderly veterans done in the seventies found that indoor UV lighting significantly increased their ability to absorb calcium from the diet. One group's living quarters contained full-spectrum lighting, which contains UV. The other group's quarters had ordinary indoor lighting, containing no UV. All of the men received approximately 200 IU per day of dietary vitamin D, but the group exposed to UV absorbed 40 percent more calcium from their diets than the group not exposed to it.[7]

Sunlight is also a recognized arthritis therapy, one that actu-

ally dates back for centuries. In a Russian study, a significant reduction in arthritis was found in miners given routine sunlight
treatments. In another study, a group of children with severe
arthritis was given cortisone, while another group was given
sunlight treatments. Relief came more slowly in the sunlight
group than in the cortisone group, but it did come; and unlike
with cortisone, there were no unwanted side effects. Resistance
to infection also increased.[8]

Early in the twentieth century, sunbathing and UV therapy
were valued as treatments not only for bone and joint conditions but for many infectious diseases, including tuberculosis.
Then, in 1938, penicillin was discovered. Sun therapy was forgotten, as drugs became big business.[9] But antibiotics have now
been so overused that they are losing their effectiveness and
may soon be obsolete. Nature herself is forcing us to return to
her own remedies, including prudent sunbathing; that is, sunbathing that is sufficient for tanning without burning.

WHAT ABOUT SKIN CANCER?

Some dermatologists, concerned about skin cancer, have gone
so far as to recommend lathering up with sunscreen every
morning, no matter what the weather, just to make sure the
skin is protected from any sunshine that might chance to fall on
it. But other experts maintain we have gone too far. Dr. Samuel
Berne, author of *Creating Your Personal Vision: A Mind-Body
Guide for Better Eyesight,* asserts that studies linking sunlight and
ultraviolet light to skin cancer were flawed. Massive doses of
UV exposure were used on animals to create skin cancer and
cataracts. The data were then extrapolated to apply to the more
normal exposures of humans to sunlight.[10]

A British and Australian study found that the incidence of
malignant melanomas (serious skin cancers) was actually higher

in office workers than in people whose lifestyles or occupations regularly exposed them to sunlight. Office workers who worked all day under fluorescent lighting had twice the normal risk of melanomas. Surprisingly, the *lowest* risk of developing skin cancer was in people whose main outdoor activity was sunbathing. These results were confirmed in two controlled studies conducted at the New York School of Medicine.[11]

Zane Kime, M.D., in a groundbreaking book called *Sunlight,* demonstrated that the sun creates free radical damage only in the presence of harmful fats and the absence of antioxidants. "Bad" fats generate free oxygen radicals, while antioxidants protect against them. The antioxidants he discussed were vitamins A, C, and E and the mineral selenium, but there are many others. Harmful fats included hydrogenated oils, refined oils, and saturated fat; in other words, the fats most common to the standard American high-fat diet.[12]

As for sunscreens, Dr. David Williams points out in the newsletter *Alternatives* that they may actually be *contributing* to skin cancer. Sunscreens encourage people to stay out in the sun longer than they otherwise would, and they prevent the formation of a protective layer of melanin on the skin. They also fail to block out the most penetrating UV wavelengths. The UV portion of the spectrum emitted by the sun includes three wavebands, UVA, UVB, and UVC. UVC wavelengths are entirely blocked by the earth's atmosphere and UVB is partially blocked, but UVA can penetrate freely to the earth. UVB is the most biologically active of the wavelengths, but UVA penetrates the most deeply. Regardless of advertising claims, says Dr. Williams, most sunscreens block out only UVB wavelengths, not the deeper-penetrating UVA wavelengths. The fact that your skin's surface doesn't burn doesn't mean you aren't being exposed to harmful rays. The melanin produced on the skin by unblocked sunshine—the suntan—is actually what protects the tissues beneath.[13] The ideal is to tan without burning. Sunscreens also contain titanium and other harmful chemicals that can be absorbed through the skin; and (contrary to popular belief) drugs applied to the skin can be more toxic than those that are ingested, because they go straight into the bloodstream without being processed in the stomach.[14] Finally, sunscreens interfere with the synthesis of vitamin D, without which ingested calcium is not incorporated into the bones but is left to settle out in the joints. As a result, sunscreens may be contributing not only to skin cancer but to arthritis and osteoporosis.

If you are worried about skin cancer from sun exposure, it's good to know that only modest exposure is necessary to avoid vitamin D deficiency. Researchers at Tufts University have shown that in the summer, minimum vitamin D requirements are met by exposure of just the hands, face, and arms for ten to fifteen minutes a day, three times a week.[15] These recommendations were made specifically for the elderly, one of the two groups most likely to need vitamin D supplementation. (The other likely group is young children. Supplements may be necessary for children if they are under six years old and live in northern industrial areas that are often cloudy.[16])

FISH OILS AND CETYL MYRISTOLEATE

Cod liver oil is good for arthritic joints not only because of its high content of vitamin D but because of its high content of essential fatty acids (EFAs). As already noted, the omega-3 fats in fatty fish block the prostaglandins that create inflammation. Fish oil capsules are available at health food stores, but therapy takes six weeks to three months to work.[17] A quicker and more effective source is cetyl myristoleate, one of the latest additions to the nutritional supplements recommended for arthritis. A com-

pound of an acid called myristoleic acid found commonly in
fish oils, whale oils, and dairy butter, cetyl myristoleate has the
same basic characteristics as the essential fatty acids, but its effects are stronger and more lasting; and the quantity required
and the period of time over which it must be taken to get an
effect are less. A large double-blind placebo-controlled study
reported that cetyl myristoleate was 63 to 87 percent effective
in relieving arthritis symptoms.

Cetyl myristoleate was discovered and isolated by Harry W.
Diehl, an employee of the National Institute of Arthritis,
Metabolism, and Digestive Diseases. Bent on finding a cure for
arthritis, he tried to induce the disease experimentally in mice
by injecting agents known to have that effect. When he was un-
able to, he concluded that the cure he was looking for was already somewhere in the animals. He eventually extracted a
compound from macerated mice identified as cetyl myristoleate. To determine whether it was the protective factor, he
injected it into rats after injecting them with a known arthritis-
inducing bacterial agent. Those receiving cetyl myristoleate had
little evidence of polyarthritis, while a control group receiving
only the bacterial agent developed severe symptoms.

Because few natural sources were known for this nutrient,
Diehl developed a method for making it in the laboratory. He
patented his discovery in 1977, receiving a use patent for
rheumatoid arthritis. But when he petitioned pharmaceutical
companies to conduct human trials, none were interested. The
discovery lay dormant for about fifteen years, until Diehl got
osteoarthritis himself. He used cetyl myristoleate on his own
condition and was cured. Word spread, and the product appeared on the market as a dietary supplement in 1991.

There have been no confirmed reports of adverse effects
from cetyl myristoleate other than mild burping as with fish

oils. The recommended course is twelve to fifteen grams daily over a one-month period.

The product is expensive, running $48 for a seventeen-day supply; but the manufacturer asserts that seventeen days is often enough to achieve significant results that can last for years, including a much better range of motion and a substantial reduction in pain.[18] In my own case, cetyl myristoleate had a noticeable beneficial effect after a few days' use. It may be ordered off the Internet at www.WholeHealthProducts.com; telephone 1-800-382-1936.

NINETEEN

Vitamins, Minerals, and Antioxidants

*For strength of nature in youth passeth over many excesses,
which are owing a man till his age. Discern of the coming on
of years, and think not to do the same things still; for age will
not be defied.*

—FRANCIS BACON,
"Of Regiment of Health"

Supplementing for vitamin and mineral deficiencies can also help relieve joint pain. Elderly people, who have a predisposition to osteoarthritis, often suffer from generalized nutrient deficiencies. Studies have shown that mineral deficits in calcium, zinc, and selenium provoke skeletal damage, and that supplementation therapies, particularly with vitamin E and the combination of vitamins B_1, B_6, and B_{12}, can exert a beneficial effect on the symptoms of degenerative joint disease.[1]

Increasing zinc intake has helped relieve symptoms particularly for rheumatoid arthritics, who have been found to have low levels of this mineral in their hair and blood. Zinc is needed along with vitamin C for maintaining normal collagen (connective) tissue, the site of disturbance in arthritis. Vitamin A also has a cooperative action with zinc. A powerful stimulant to the immune system, zinc is generally deficient in the American diet due to the overprocessing of foods.

Calcium and magnesium are also particularly important for joint health. Calcium is essential for maintaining healthy bones, joints, muscles, and ligaments; but without magnesium, calcium won't be incorporated into these structures properly and can build up as extraskeletal calcification in the soft tissues and joints. Magnesium is also a natural pain reliever. Low levels of magnesium increase nerve cell excitability and pain.[2] Low magnesium levels can result from high protein diets, which contain excess phosphorus. Phosphorus binds up magnesium and makes it unavailable for use. Extra magnesium supplementation is therefore recommended. Magnesium also helps relieve muscle spasms and protects the heart against stress. To reduce leg cramping, calcium supplements may help too.

Boron is another mineral that is important for the retention of calcium in the bones.[3] Other minerals necessary for preserving the joints and bones include manganese and iron. Potassium (along with vitamins C and B_6) helps reduce pain and inflammation by decreasing local fluid levels. Natural sources of potassium include oranges, bananas, figs, raisins, dates, and nuts.

The importance of sulfur for the bones was discussed in chapter 16. Besides being found in MSM and glucosamine sulfate, it can be obtained from garlic, onions, Brussels sprouts, and cabbage.

Copper is also required for healthy joints. Copper helps reduce the pain and inflammation of osteoarthritis because superoxide dismutase (SOD), a powerful free radical scavenger within the joint, depends on it. Copper is necessary for normal metabolism and tissue health but cannot be synthesized by the body. It must be obtained from outside sources. Unfortunately, the copper content of food is declining due to serious soil depletion.[4]

ANOTHER LOOK AT THE COPPER BRACELET

The copper requirement for healthy joints may explain the popularity of another folk remedy for arthritic complaints, the copper bracelet. Enthusiastic claims like these have been made for it: "I have worn my copper bracelet for one year and it is the best thing for my arthritis." "Since wearing my copper bracelet I have cut down on taking aspirin and many days I am pain free and able to do my job."[5] Wild as these claims sound, there is evidence in their support. Copper has actually been used for thousands of years to treat inflammation.

The subject was heavily researched by two American professors, Dr. H. Dollwet from the University of Akron and Dr. J. Sorenson from the University of Arkansas, who found many historical uses of copper as an anti-inflammatory agent and as a promoter of general well-being.[6] The world's oldest medical text, the Egyptian Ebers papyrus, recommended pulverized copper to treat inflammation of various sorts. In medieval Germany, Paracelsus prescribed copper for a variety of ills. In 1939, German physician Werner Hangarter reported that Finnish copper miners were free of joint inflammation, although rheumatism was widespread in Finland. Dr. Hangarter successfully treated patients suffering from rheumatic fever, rheumatoid arthritis, and neck and back problems with copper compounds. Copper chelates were used as arthritis drugs from the 1940s to the 1950s in France and Germany, but interest in this therapy waned with the introduction of the corticosteroids.

Like natural remedies in general, the copper bracelet is not a popular subject for research because it cannot be patented as a medical device or generate funding for research projects. But at least one researcher has put this folk remedy to the test. Dr. Ray Walker of the University of Newcastle in Australia studied three hundred arthritis sufferers. Group I, who had previously worn copper bracelets, were asked not to wear them for a month. Group II, who had never worn the bracelets, were given two indistinguishable ones, one made of copper and the other a placebo made of aluminum. They were instructed to wear each one for a month. Group I reported that their symptoms were significantly worse when not wearing the bracelets, while Group II reported feeling best during the month they wore the bracelets that proved to be the copper ones.[7]

Dr. Walker attributed these effects to absorption of trace amounts of copper from the bracelets. When copper comes in contact with the skin, it forms chelates with compounds of human sweat and is thus absorbed through the skin.

An alternative theory for the effectiveness of the copper bracelet is that it acts as a battery that stores and returns electromagnetic energy to the body. This was the explanation of Indian adepts who recommended wearing pure metal jewelry for health and strength.

On that theory, handcrafted copper bracelets are more therapeutic than the machine-made variety. The pressure applied by machine deforms the microscopic crystal lattice of the metal, making it rigid and brittle. Excellent handcrafted copper bracelets are available at a reasonable price from Sergio Lub Handcrafted Copper Bracelets in Martinez, California, telephone 925-229-3600.

ANTIOXIDANTS

Other nutrients reduce pain by reducing free radical formation. These are the antioxidants, including vitamins E and C, beta-carotene, selenium (found in garlic and onions, among other sources), pycnogenol, bioflavonoids, coenzyme Q10, and alpha lipoic acid. Also having anti-inflammatory and antioxidant effects are boron, zinc, copper, manganese, pantothenic acid, methionine, superoxide dismutase, proteolytic enzymes, L-phenylalanine, tryptophan, and sulfur (cysteine).

That laundry list is too long to take individually, but there are good combination products on the market that allow intake of many nutrients in one capsule. One mentioned earlier that is designed specifically for arthritis is Arth-X Plus by Trace Minerals Research in Roy, Utah. It contains glucosamine sulfate and trace minerals among a long list of other nutrients and herbs.

GREEN DRINKS AND CHLOROPHYLL

Another way to get a range of nutrients in one product is with "green" drinks, including "Green Magma," "Barley Green," "Kyo-Green," and "Green Radiance." Deep-green plants are constantly exposed to the high-energy rays of the sun. Plants transform these rays into chlorophyll, an antioxidant that protects them from oxidative damage. Chlorophyll is an excellent cleanser and has anti-inflammatory properties. Besides in deep-green vegetables, you can get chlorophyll as tablets or in alfalfa tea.

The benefits of chlorophyll on arthritis were illustrated in a case cited by Julian Whitaker, M.D., involving a patient who had had severe rheumatoid arthritis for about four years. She was taking the toxic drug Plaquenil, and prednisone had been recommended next; but she had declined. Instead, Dr. Whitaker started her on large doses of a green drink called "GREENS+," along with antioxidants, glucosamine sulfate, fish oil supplements, and flaxseed oil. Meanwhile, the patient gradually reduced her dosage of Plaquenil. In two weeks, her symptoms had significantly lessened and the movement in her hands had significantly increased.[8]

ANTIOXIDANTS AND OTHER NUTRITIONAL
REMEDIES FOR FIBROMYALGIA

Antioxidants are of particular benefit to fibromyalgia sufferers. Vitamin E has been shown to benefit them dramatically in some cases. Another antioxidant found to help in cases of both fibromyalgia and arthritis is pycnogenol, a natural compound extracted from the bark of the French maritime pine tree and grape seeds.[9] Pycnogenol reactivates damaged collagen by binding to collagen fibers and realigning them to a more youthful undamaged form, quenches free radicals, reduces inflammation, and boosts the immune system.

Fibromyalgia symptoms have also been relieved by a combination of malic acid (magnesium maleate) and boswellia, an herb used traditionally in India. Although malic acid alone can help fibromyalgia pain, the combination is more effective. One downside is that the supplements have to be taken every six hours or so. If they are stopped, the pain returns, indicating that they are still only masking pain; but they do avoid the side effects of conventional drugs and are more effective than ordinary analgesics.

A protocol that has been known to work on fibromyalgia when all else fails is one produced by a multilevel marketing company called Life Plus, using products called Lyprinex (consisting of special oils) and Proanthonols (strong antioxidants). Both are taken at very high doses the first month, making the first month's treatment quite expensive (around $300); but in subsequent months, the dosage and cost are reduced.

SAMe FOR ARTHRITIS AND FIBROMYALGIA

A new addition to the nutritional supplements available for relieving the pain of arthritis and fibromyalgia is S-adenosylmethionine (SAMe). Sold in Europe as an antidepressant drug, SAMe is the activated form of methionine, an amino acid. In a crossover study reported in the *American Journal of Medicine* comparing SAMe and a placebo in the treatment of fibromyalgia, the number of trigger points and painful anatomic sites decreased in fibromyalgia sufferers using SAMe but not the placebo. Scores for depression also significantly improved on SAMe but not the placebo. The researchers concluded that SAMe is a safe and effective therapy in the management of fibromyalgia.[10]

A number of studies have also established the effectiveness of SAMe in the treatment of arthritic complaints in general. A review of research in the *American Journal of Medicine* concluded that the results of extensive clinical trials involving about 22,000 patients with osteoarthritis support the clinical safety and effectiveness of SAMe administration. Experimental investigations suggest that SAMe exerts analgesic and anti-inflammatory activities and stimulates the synthesis of proteoglycans, without the side effects on the gastrointestinal tract and other organs incurred with NSAIDs. While the intensity of the therapeutic activity of SAMe against osteoarthritis was similar to that of NSAIDs, its tolerability was higher. The researchers proposed SAMe as the prototype of a new class of safe treatment for osteoarthritis.[11]

In Switzerland, a randomized double-blind multicenter clinical trial was conducted to compare the effectiveness and tolerance of SAMe and the NSAID ibuprofen in 150 patients with hip or knee osteoarthritis. Both remedies were given orally, 400 mg three times daily for thirty days. SAMe was found to be slightly more active in pain management than ibuprofen, and side effects were substantially less frequent.[12]

A Scandinavian placebo–controlled study reported in 1991

found that SAMe reduced clinical disease activity, pain, fatigue, morning stiffness, and depression.[13]

In a long-term multicenter open trial in Germany, the efficacy and tolerance of SAMe were studied for twenty-four months in 108 patients with osteoarthritis of the knee, hip, and spine. The patients received 600 mg of SAMe daily for the first two weeks and 400 mg daily thereafter. SAMe showed good clinical effectiveness and was well tolerated, with improvement of clinical symptoms already evident after the first weeks of treatment and continuing up to the end of the study. SAMe also relieved the depressive feelings often associated with osteoarthritis. Side effects were minor and disappeared by the last six months of treatment.[14] Gastrointestinal upset, the most serious side effect reported for SAMe, is significantly less frequent than with NSAIDs and is attributed to its action on the head (as in motion sickness) rather than on stomach prostaglandins (as with NSAIDs).

Researchers have concluded that SAMe, like glucosamine and chondroitin sulfate, may go beyond the symptoms of arthritis to actually slowing the disease itself. If so, these nutrients represent a revolutionary breakthrough in the treatment of the disease.[15]

TWENTY

The Hormone Connection

The doctor of the future will give no medicine but will interest his patients in the care of the human frame, in diet, and in the cause and prevention of disease.

—THOMAS EDISON

That hormones play a role in arthritis remains controversial but is suggested by circumstantial evidence, including the suspicious facts that RA is largely a women's disease, striking three times as many women as men; seven out of eight fibromyalgia sufferers are women, most commonly in their mid-thirties or in menopause; many women develop osteoarthritis during menopause; and pregnant and menopausal women are particularly prone to developing carpal tunnel syndrome.[1]

Researchers at the Baylor University Medical Center in Dallas pursued a hormonal lead for rheumatoid arthritis after observing that pregnant women with the disease went into remission for the length of their pregnancies. When they treated women with RA with weekly injections of estrogen and progesterone, the women's conditions improved dramatically by both subjective and objective measures.[2]

Estrogen and progesterone need to be in balance for the body to function normally, but many women have too much or too little of one or the other. The trick is figuring out which hormone needs to be supplemented. In arthritis, the likely culprit is a lack of progesterone. This statement is borne out by the fact that estradiol, a type of estrogen found in pharmaceutical estrogens, has been found to promote arthritis pain.[3] One reason may be that estrogen causes edema (water retention), which crowds the joints and presses on the nerves, contributing to carpal tunnel syndrome and other joint pains. Herbal remedies, including licorice root, dong quai, and alfalfa, have been shown to block the negative effects of estrogen on the joints.[4]

Natural progesterone cream has also been found to be effective in relieving arthritis pain when rubbed into painful joints over a period of time.[5] Progesterone is a precursor from which other hormones are made. Pregnenolone is another natural hormone precursor shown to help in some types of arthritis.[6] Pregnenolone helps keep hormone levels in balance.

NATURAL ALTERNATIVES TO PHARMACEUTICAL HORMONES

Besides contributing to joint pain, pharmaceutical estrogen can have other unwanted side effects. The most popular pharmaceutical combination of hormone replacement therapy is Provera (synthetic progesterone) and Premarin (estrogen derived from mare's urine). Side effects listed for Premarin in the *Physician's Desk Reference* include not only water retention but PMS-like symptoms; breast tenderness, enlargement, and secretion; nausea, vomiting, abdominal cramps, and bloating; skin and eye sensitivities; headaches, dizziness, and depression; weight gain; bleeding between periods or missed periods; changes in libido (sex drive); and enlargement of uterine fibroid tumors.

Even worse side effects, however, are attributed to synthetic progesterone (Provera). They include water retention, nausea, insomnia, jaundice, mental depression, fever, masculinization, weight changes, breast tenderness, abdominal cramping, anxiety, irritability, and allergic reactions. Fluid retention can exacerbate asthma, migraines, epilepsy, and heart and kidney problems.[7]

For women who feel they need hormones but want to minimize the side effects and risks of the prescription versions, estrogen and progesterone are available as natural hormone creams derived from plants. John Lee, M.D., of Sebastopol, California, showed in his bestselling 1996 book *What Your Doctor May Not Tell You About Menopause* that natural progesterone cream (Pro-Gest) is more effective than pharmaceutical estrogen in reversing bone loss, and avoids its side effects. The sterols of plants such as soybeans and yams are the basis from which many cheap, commercially available hormones are made. Soybeans and yams are good food sources of natural estrogen and progesterone, as are fennel, celery, parsley, nuts, whole grains, and apples.

NATURAL PROGESTERONE AND CARPAL TUNNEL SYNDROME

Natural progesterone cream can relieve not only arthritic pain but carpal tunnel syndrome. The condition begins with tingling and numbness in the fingers and wrist joints, especially at night, progressing to persistent pain and aching in the hands and arms. As already noted, pregnant and menopausal women are particularly affected by it. Conventional treatment includes wrist splints, pain relievers, surgery, and avoidance of unnecessary repetitive stress. Alternative practitioners also recommend acupuncture, chiropractic, massage, ultrasound, yoga, and homeopathy to help relieve pain by increasing circulation. But while these measures treat the symptoms, for many women the underlying cause is the little-suspected one of hormone imbalance. Women who have had carpal tunnel syndrome for years have been cured in a matter of weeks simply by applying natural progesterone cream to their wrists.

PERSONAL EXPERIENCE

This approach worked for me, allowing me to throw away the wrist splints I had worn nightly for seventeen years, ever since pregnancy with my first child. I have to admit to being somewhat sporadic in my intake of nutritional supplements, but I apply my natural hormone creams religiously (except for three days out of the month, the minimum abstention recommended to allow the hormone receptor sites to resensitize to the hormones). I attribute to natural progesterone cream the reversal not only of my carpal tunnel syndrome but of a prolapsed uterus. I added natural estrogen cream later to counteract hot flashes, for which I found it quite satisfactory. In my case, the "side effects" of these creams were only good ones, including increased sex drive and a reduction in stress level.

The progesterone cream that works best for me is Pro-Gest by Transitions for Health in Portland, Oregon (telephone 800-861-5009). I have tried other brands and only this one counteracts the prolapse in my uterus, which returns after about three days without it. For natural estrogen, I like Ostaderm by Bezwecken in Beaverton, Oregon (available from the Golden Cabinet, telephone 631-725-5720). For a fuller discussion of natural hormone replacement, see Ellen Brown and Lynne Walker, *Menopause and Estrogen*.[8]

PROGESTERONE, VITAMIN B$_6$, AND RHEUMATIC PAIN

The hormone connection could also help explain why vitamin B$_6$ (pyridoxine) works on some cases of carpal tunnel syndrome and other rheumatic pains, since vitamin B$_6$ is known to stimulate the production of progesterone in the body. Vitamin B$_6$ has been found to relieve tingling in the hands and arms; cramps in the legs; swelling in hands, fingers, and feet; and pain in finger joints and shoulders.

Vitamin B$_6$ therapy for rheumatism was pioneered by Dr. John Ellis, who successfully treated hundreds of patients with it and reported that responses were often "spectacular." For the therapy to work, he found that a balanced diet was required along with 50 to 100 mg of vitamin B$_6$ daily.

JOINT PAIN AND THYROID DEFICIENCY

Another hormone imbalance linked to aching, stiffness, and weakness of muscles and joints is a deficiency of thyroid hormone. This problem, too, is one to which women are particularly prone. Besides muscle and joint pain, symptoms of depressed thyroid function include constipation, frequent colds, dry skin, dry hair, brittle nails, cold feet, and fatigue.

If medical testing indicates a thyroid hormone deficiency, a daily oral dose of Armour Thyroid (natural thyroid hormone) can eliminate these symptoms. There are also natural thyroid boosters, including iodine and vitamin B$_1$. Using natural iodine sources such as kelp is better than relying on iodized salt, which can unduly increase sodium intake.[9]

A simple home alternative for testing your thyroid function is to shake down a thermometer before going to sleep and place it next to the bed. When you wake up, before getting up, tuck it under your armpit and leave it there for ten minutes. If the temperature averages less than 97.8 degrees F, you are likely to have an underactive thyroid.[10] If you suspect thyroid problems, consult a qualified health practitioner.

Part 4

~

REGULATION
THERAPIES

TWENTY-ONE

The First Regulation Therapy: Exercise

Health is the vital principle of bliss,
And exercise of health.

—JAMES THOMSON,
"The Castle of Indolence" (1748)

Unlike supplementation therapies, which work by supplying miss-ing nutrients, regulation therapies work by correcting malfunctions in body systems and reestablishing the flow of blood and energy to areas that have been blocked for a long period of time. Besides practitioner-based techniques for achieving these results, there is an essential therapy for reestablishing blood flow to the joints that can be done at home in your spare time, without a practitioner and without charge. This is exercise, something arthritics may resist just because it hurts their joints but that remains essential for recovery. Ways around the pain problem will be suggested in this chapter, after a look at the fundamental importance of the endeavor.

THE CRITICAL IMPORTANCE
OF EXERCISING THE JOINTS

For cells to grow and repair themselves, they need a supply of nutrients and oxygen and a means of eliminating waste products. Most cells are serviced for these purposes by a continuous supply of blood, but joint cartilage has no blood supply. Instead, cartilage cells get their nutrients and dispose of their waste products through the synovial fluid (the fluid in the joint). The joint works like a sponge, squeezing waste-laden fluid out and drawing nutrient-laden fluid in. If the sponge isn't squeezed, the cartilage degenerates from lack of nutrients. In addition to carrying nutrients in and waste products out, the synovial fluid lubricates the joints. Those functions all depend on mechanical movement through exercise, which keeps the joint cells fed.[1]

If exercise is avoided, the cartilage surrounding the joint can begin to break down. The body responds by forming new cartilage and bone at the site. Whether this is an attempt to replace what is lost or is an effort at immobilization, the eventual result is an entire crusting over of the joint. At that point, natural methods for reversing the damage are too late.

Restricting motion of any body part also causes the muscles to weaken and deteriorate. In the legs, the blood may pool in the veins, causing the legs to swell. The bones lose calcium and grow thin. Exercise is necessary not only to maintain joint flexibility but to strengthen the muscles around them. Stronger muscles reduce wear on cartilage and bone and help reduce pain.

Exercise also helps relieve tension, which can cause the pain of fibromyalgia and other rheumatic diseases. When sedentary people fail to release tension through exercise and other normal outlets, it stays in the muscles, contracting them and making them stiff. Pain in the joints can also be the result of tension in the muscles. To fix the problem in these cases, you need to restore the normal length, strength, and flexibility of the dysfunctioning muscles by stretching and exercise.[2]

Exercise not only delays the progression of arthritis but can actually reverse damage to the joints. This has been demonstrated in studies in which damage to the joint cartilage of arthritic rabbits was reduced just by moving the animals' joints.[3] The same therapy works for humans. The notoriously limited capacity of immobilized joints to heal or regenerate led Canadian researcher R. B. Salter to the concept of continuous passive motion of synovial joints—moving the joints on a machine that did the work. Since then, scientific investigations involving animals and humans have confirmed that merely moving the joints mechanically stimulates the growth of articular cartilage and accelerates the healing of articular tissues.[4]

THE CATCH: ARTHRITIS MAKES EXERCISE PAINFUL

The advice of physical therapists is to move every joint in all its natural directions daily, but arthritics are liable to avoid this exercise because it hurts. To mask the pain of arthritic joints long enough to do the needed exercise, physical therapists sometimes give painkillers, including narcotic painkillers such as codeine; cortisone and its derivatives (e.g., prednisone), which reduce inflammation and its resulting pain; and antihypertensive drugs such as reserpine and propranolol, which block the effects of the adrenaline production that results in inflammation.[5] The downside of this approach is that the drugs have side effects; and when you are feeling no pain, you can overstress the joints and do more harm than good.

HYDROTHERAPY

One side-effect-free option is to warm up your joints first in water. Hot water increases blood flow to the joints and relieves muscle pain. While you are submerged in your bath or pool, you can exercise the joints at the same time. Water frees them from the effects of gravity and the weight of the limbs and allows them to move more easily. Twenty to thirty minutes in the pool is good, or fifteen in the Jacuzzi. While in a pool you can also practice walking or jogging. Water gymnastic exercises are excellent. You'll find you can get your joints to move in the water in ways they won't move on dry land. If water exercises produce pain, it may be not from stress on the joint but from unused muscle groups, which sometimes take time to get back in shape. Go slow and use pain as a guide. As your joints gradually regain their strength and flexibility in the water, they will also work better out of it.

HOT OR COLD?

Both hot and cold water have their uses for arthritic joints. Heat increases blood flow, improves the delivery of nutrients, and aids in relaxation. It can be administered not only in the Jacuzzi or sauna but locally with hot water bottles, electric heating pads, or hot towels.

If your pain is caused by acute inflammation, however, heat can make it worse by causing tissue swelling and bringing in additional white blood cells that contribute to the inflammatory process; and generalized heat, as in a hot tub, can increase the demands on the heart if it is too hot or too sustained.

Cold applications have the opposite effect. The blood vessels contract, blood flow is reduced, the inflammatory process is slowed, and swelling is reduced. Cold water also improves muscle tone. Cold can be applied with cold towels, ice packs, or in a cold water hip bath.

The cold water hip bath has to be experienced to be appreciated. While it sounds daunting, it is actually an invigorating experience that can become addicting. Fill the tub with enough cold water to cover the hips, then sit in it. Splash the water all over your body and rub vigorously. As long as you keep moving, you won't feel chilled. Begin with the arms, then splash water on the sides, back, and stomach. The abdominal area is particularly important. The congested liver retains heat, and cold water helps to decongest it. Five minutes in the tub is sufficient.

Then there is the ice pack treatment. Doctors at the Germantown Medical Center in Pennsylvania found that patients with RA were able to cut their medicine intake in half by applying baggies full of ice to their knees for twenty minutes three times a day. All twenty-four patients in the study reported relief of symptoms. The procedure was to fill two baggies with six ice cubes and a quart of cold water each and hold them firmly above and below the knee for twenty minutes. Any discomfort faded after about five minutes, when an anesthetic effect set in. Oddly, the patients said they experienced relief in both knees though the baggies were applied to only one. The researchers attributed this phenomenon to an increase in circulating endorphins produced by the cold. Endorphins are natural pain-relievers and sleep-inducers.

Another alternative that is inexpensive, comfortable, and effective is to wrap a large pack of frozen peas or corn kernels (which are flexible and conform to the body) in a thin towel and apply to inflamed areas.

For arthritic hands and feet, try placing those extremities first in hot water, then in cold water, alternating half a dozen times over the space of about forty minutes. This will increase blood flow to the area and aid healing, while at the same time relieving pain.[6]

EXERCISE AND FIBROMYALGIA

Exercise isn't easy for fibromyalgia victims, since one of the predominant symptoms of this debilitating condition is fatigue.

Sufferers have a hard time just getting out of bed. If they can bring themselves to do vigorous exercise, however, it is worth the effort. Exercise produces endorphins; it increases blood flow to the muscles; and it increases levels of serotonin and growth hormone, two substances that seem to be deficient in people with fibromyalgia and that restore muscle fitness and improve pain tolerance.[7]

CAUTIONS WHEN EXERCISING

Be sure to warm up and stretch the muscles before working them, since exercise done improperly can actually make arthritis worse. Tight muscles can cause the joints to move in unnatural ways that wind up straining and damaging them. Shorter, more frequent periods of exercise are better than a vigorous once-a-week competition in which the will to win can overrule the body's warning signals to ease up and go slow. Do the exercise correctly, don't exercise when your joints are inflamed, and don't overstress them. You are liable to experience serious pain only *after* the excess stress has been imposed, so listen to more subtle warnings that you are overdoing it and quit while you're ahead. It also pays to invest in a pair of good shock-absorbing shoes.

TWENTY-TWO

Manual Manipulation: Massage, Chiropractic, Reflexology, and Craniosacral Therapy

Sweet is pleasure after pain.

—JOHN DRYDEN,
"Alexander's Feast" (1687)

The naturopathic explanation for arthritic and rheumatic disorders of all types is that metabolic wastes and other toxic substances build up in the blood, causing the blood to thicken and the circulation to slow. The tissues become asphyxiated from lack of oxygen, causing the muscles to contract. The result is rheumatic and arthritic pain.

That explanation throws light on the relief that massage and other forms of manual manipulation can give to distressed joints: they help activate the circulation by channeling wastes for excretion. Manual manipulation ranges from simple massage to craniosacral therapy, a sophisticated technique that is particularly helpful for fibromyalgia sufferers.

MASSAGE

Massage, the oldest known form of physical therapy, has something of a bad name today, perhaps from its association with "massage parlors." But its therapeutic effects can exceed those of the more reputable drug options; and unless you count the occasional raised eyebrow of a spouse, they come without side effects. Massage causes the muscles to relax and improves nutrition to the joints and surrounding tissues by increasing the flow of fluids to them. It also stretches tendons and muscles, improving their motion; and it acts as a natural sedative, improving sleep without the hangover-like side effects of the pharmaceutical versions.

Massage was often combined by the ancients with hot baths and rubbing of the body with oil. Today, liniments that relieve pain by acting as counterirritants may be rubbed into the skin. Methyl salicylate, the active ingredient in oil of wintergreen and sweet birch oil, is a popular remedy.

REFLEXOLOGY

Reflexology is a technique that evolved out of an earlier European system known as zone therapy, involving pressure on and massage of "reflex" points on the feet and hands. Reflexology is now practiced by nearly 25,000 practitioners worldwide and is the number one alternative therapy in Denmark.

Reflexologists say that a life energy, or vital force, circulates between the organs of the body, permeating every tissue and cell. This energy is divided into a number of zones which terminate in the feet and hands. Toxins drain by gravity to the extremities. By breaking up painful gritty areas or crystal deposits there, the reflexologist frees up the entire energy zone connected to them. Pressure and massage of the reflex points on the extremities dissipate energy blocks, break down crystalline structure, stimulate the circulatory and lymphatic systems, and encourage the release of toxins. The body is thus stimulated to heal itself.[1]

When I tried this therapy, the most painful point on my feet turned out to be that reflexing to my hip. After an hour-long reflexology treatment that was limited to my feet, my hip actually felt more limber and free. And the therapy itself was sheer pleasure.

CHIROPRACTIC ADJUSTMENT

Chiropractors maintain that some cases diagnosed as arthritis (particularly osteoarthritis) are actually the result of misalignment or "subluxation" of the vertebrae and joints. In cases of this type, chiropractic adjustment has resulted in complete relief of symptoms.[2]

In a book called *Natural Relief for Arthritis,* Carol Keough reports the case of a woman diagnosed with a bad case of degenerative osteoarthritis. Her symptoms disappeared simply after having ten chiropractic adjustments and taking a variety of dietary supplements aimed at replacing missing nutrients.[3]

In my own case, chiropractic adjustment helped with a problem of unequal leg lengths evidently resulting from a tightness in the hips that threw their balance off. I was told that the longer leg shoved further into the joint, putting added pressure on it when I walked. Adjustment helped correct this disparity, relieving the pressure on the joint and the resulting pain.

ROLFING

Rolfing is a form of deep muscle massage developed by Dr. Ida Rolf, a biochemist, to eliminate her own arthritis. She discovered that stretching the fascial tissues (thin sheets of connective tissue holding muscles, joints, and organs together) can change the underlying conditions causing arthritic disturbances by repositioning the body in alignment with gravity. She observed that many cases diagnosed as arthritis reflect only a shortened or displaced muscle or ligament resulting from a prior trauma to the area.[4]

One drawback of Rolfing is that some recipients find it to be quite painful. In my own case it was not, but what I enjoyed more and found to be more effective was a gentler technique based on similar principles called craniosacral therapy.

CRANIOSACRAL THERAPY

A painless form of manual manipulation that is particularly helpful for relieving fibromyalgia and other rheumatic pain, craniosacral therapy has its roots in cranial osteopathy, a system developed in the nineteenth century by Andrew Taylor Still, M.D. Dr. Still emphasized the importance of maintaining normal blood and nerve flow and the release of blockages in the energy patterns of the body. Cranial osteopathy is a nonforceful manual technique that helps the body dissolve the strain patterns created by blunt trauma during injury. It also improves the flow of nutrients to tissues and organs, boosts the immune system, and assists the elimination of waste products through the lymphatic system. Craniosacral therapy is a technique taught by the International Association of Health Care Practitioners in Palm Beach Gardens, Florida, headed by John Upledger, D.O.

My introduction to this technique came from Dr. Oram Miller, a chiropractor in San Diego. He observed that my entire body was torqued, probably from when a car wheel ran across my pelvic bones at seventeen. This twist had thrown my hips out of alignment, resulting in the uneven leg lengths observed by my chiropractor. A series of craniosacral adjustments helped by gently untwisting my body, relieving the pressure on my hip from the longer leg.

CRANIOSACRAL THERAPY AND THE
STRAIN PATTERNS OF FIBROMYALGIA

While he was treating me, Dr. Miller gave this interesting discourse on the technique and on the cause and appropriate treatment of fibromyalgia:

The premise behind craniosacral therapy is that there is a motion in every human from birth to death, twenty-four hours a day, originating in the head and spreading gently through the entire body like a fluid wave. This motion is automatic; it goes on even if you hold your breath. It is necessary for life and is termed the primary respiratory mechanism, to distinguish it from breathing. The conventional view of the skull is that its sutures (the lines between the bones) are fused by adulthood, making the skull one solid immovable structure. However, research conducted by Dr. Upledger and his colleagues, using special stains on fresh sections of skull suture bones obtained at surgery, showed that these sutures are not ossified in adults but are filled with a rich network of trabecular fibers of fascia, nerve endings, blood vessels, and cells. The bones of the head thus have the capacity to move relative to each other, however slightly.

The structures of the head, including the bones and meninges (coverings) of the brain, have been found to move approximately eight to twelve times per minute. This motion, which is a little slower than breathing, is in response to a natural change in the pressure of the cerebrospinal fluid. Cranial osteopaths are taught to monitor this motion and determine if it has been jammed, compressed, or contorted in any way from previous injury. Since most injuries are whole-body in nature, these strain patterns can affect the patient anywhere in the musculoskeletal system. Cranial techniques involve locating and releasing these patterns.

The craniosacral system consists of the brain and spinal cord, the cerebrospinal fluid bathing them, the surrounding membranes enclosing them, and the bones of the spine and skull. Craniosacral therapy works with the rhythm that results in the cranial system from the increase and decrease in volume of the cerebrospinal fluid. The craniosacral rhythm causes the skull bones to move in a slight but predictable way. Restrictions to this movement can result in disease. Such restrictions result from injury, inflexibility of the joints of the cranium and spine, or dysfunctions in other parts of the body. By releasing these restrictions and restoring function, craniosacral therapy can be of benefit in cases of muscular rheumatism such as fibromyalgia, along with a range of other conditions.

The craniosacral motion needs to be as free, balanced, and symmetrical as possible for optimum health. Whenever there is a traumatic blow, such as a fall, this motion becomes jammed and compressed in the head or body and is prevented from fully expressing itself. This can cause a host of medical problems, including chronic pain syndromes, arthritis, jaw pain, middle ear infection, depression, and fibromyalgia. These strain patterns stay with the person for decades afterward, one injury strain pattern winding up layered upon another, weaving into a latticework within the connective tissue structures of the body—the muscles, joints, ligaments and tendons. These are the patients who years later say, "I don't know what I did, Doc, but I bent over to pick up a towel and my back gave out." The problem is actually traceable to earlier injuries.

Often the original injury is an auto accident. Force vectors enter the body and get lost in the tissues at the time of the accident. The body dissolves these force vectors in the minutes, hours, and days that follow. They go in as kinetic energy and come out as thermal energy. Though much of the energy of a car accident can go through the body and out the other side, some of it stays for decades. Unless the person gets evaluated and treated by a practitioner of cranial technique within days or weeks of an accident to get these subliminal patterns out, they will be carried around for years. According to Dr. Upledger, the energy gets locked in the tissues as "energy cysts." Cranial manipulation breaks up these energy cysts in a very gentle way. One of the benefits of craniosacral therapy over more forceful techniques of manipulation is that the inherent healing capacity of the body is acknowledged.

Treatment lasts twenty to thirty minutes and involves the whole body (not just the cranium, or skull, as the name implies). The practitioner has the patient lie on her back, then simply places his hands under the spine or other part of the body that is restricted, allowing the force of gravity to release tension naturally. The fascia are also very gently manipulated by a light touch on the skin through the clothing.

"I don't heal people," says Dr. Miller. "I catalyze their bodies to do the healing and releasing, but only at the pace they're ready for. I wait and let the patient's body unwind at its natural pace. When the suppleness and freedom of internal motion are restored, the cranial motion becomes much more free of its own accord. That's what I'm waiting for."

For a craniosacral therapist in your area, call the Cranial Academy in Indianapolis (telephone 317-594-0411), or check the website of the Upledger Institute, www.upledger.com. Dr. Miller can be reached by e-mail at oram@home.com.

TWENTY-THREE

Acupuncture

The superior doctor prevents illness; the mediocre doctor cures imminent illness; the inferior doctor treats illness.

—CHINESE PROVERB

The regulation therapy that is most well accepted among doctors today is acupuncture. Fifty percent of 780 doctors responding to a 1995 survey used acupuncture in their practice, mostly to control pain, treat arthritis, and for detoxification programs.[1] Acupuncture treatment is popular in hospitals for pain relief, and training programs are widely available for M.D.s. Nationally, an estimated 12,000 nonphysicians also practice it. Twenty-four states currently either license or certify acupuncturists, and more than thirty accredited schools nationwide offer three- and four-year master's level programs for non-M.D. acupuncturists.

The popularity of this Far Eastern technique is surprising, since acupuncture is based on a totally different paradigm from that of Western medicine. The aim of acupuncture is to correct imbalances in an energy field Western medicine doesn't even recognize. The diagnosis "osteoarthritis of the knee" does not exist in traditional Chinese medicine. The closest translation is "the knee area energy is blocked."[2] Acknowledging that acupuncture works means accepting that the body is criss-crossed with a system of energy pathways that can be stimulated with tiny needles.[3]

Not long ago, sticking the body with pins was derided by Western doctors as a form of voodoo. Then in 1971, columnist James Reston wrote in the *New York Times* about an emergency appendectomy he underwent in China, in which anesthesia was successfully induced using nothing more than a few carefully placed metal needles.[4] In 1974, the National Institutes of Health approved the study of acupuncture for the possible management of chronic pain caused by cancer, neuralgia, and arthritis. Since then, the technique has gained wide acceptance among doctors and hospitals in the United States. In November 1997, a consensus panel convened by the National Institutes of Health concluded there is clear evidence that acupuncture is effective for relieving pain in a variety of situations, including postoperative and chemotherapy nausea and vomiting, nausea of pregnancy, and postoperative dental pain.

THE APPROACH

Acupuncture, while new to Western medicine, goes back more than two thousand years in China, where it is used for pain relief, anesthesia, and in the treatment of various ailments including arthritis. Traditional Chinese medical techniques include not only acupuncture but acupressure, herbal remedies, and qi gong (a discipline that combines breathing, meditation, and relaxation techniques to enhance the flow of energy through the body). The goal of these techniques is to regulate body function by treating the whole person, enhancing the body's innate healing abilities through a combination of herbs, food, exercise, breathing, massage, and stimulation of the body's own healing energies.

Acupuncture stimulates the energy needed for healing by insertion of a number of very fine metal needles into the skin at specially designated points. There are about eight hundred traditional acupuncture points, arranged along fourteen lines, or meridians, running from head to foot down the body. The points of insertion may or may not be near the affected organ of the body, but they correspond to a line of energy that travels to the affected area. The needles vary in length from one-half inch to several inches and are twirled and vibrated in specific ways. A battery-powered device may also be used to provide electrical stimulation through the needles. Acupuncture may be combined with moxabustion, the burning of leaves of moxa (Chinese wormwood). Chinese studies suggest that this herb stimulates the acupuncture points and hastens healing.

The traditional explanation for why acupuncture works is based on Taoist philosophy, which says that good health depends on a free circulation of *qi* (life force energy) through the meridians or main channels of flow to the organs of the body. This force is controlled by two forms of energy, yin (negative) and yang (positive). Energy flow along a meridian can be impeded by toxic accumulations, diseased organs, or stress (physical, chemical, or emotional). Illness in other organs along the meridian may then result. Piercing appropriate points on the meridian stimulates the flow of *qi,* clears blockages, and corrects imbalances.

The problem for Western researchers is that *qi* isn't measurable or detectable by conventional methods. Alternative explanations have therefore been proposed. One is that the needles stimulate the nervous system to release endorphins or other naturally occurring chemicals and hormones that affect mood, health, and pain perception. Western researchers have found that the acupuncture points correspond to points on the skin having less electrical resistance than other skin areas. Where skin resistance is low, a greater current of the energy necessary for healing is transmitted.

ACUPUNCTURE AND ARTHRITIS

A number of studies have demonstrated acupuncture's effectiveness on arthritis. In one study reported in the *Bulletin of the New York Academy of Medicine,* 109 people with arthritis of different types received acupuncture treatments. Eighty-one experienced either complete or partial improvement over a six-month period.[5]

In a University of Maryland study reported in 1997, fifty-eight patients with moderate-to-severe knee osteoarthritis were randomized either to receive traditional Chinese acupuncture twice weekly for eight weeks along with their usual medical therapy, or to remain on medical therapy alone. Pain and disability measures were similar in the two groups. Significant improvement in pain and disability scores was found for patients receiving acupuncture when assessed at four, eight, and twelve weeks, while no significant improvement was reported in the control group. Dr. Marc Hochberg, who headed the study, observed that acupuncture is widely used in Asian countries to treat arthritis, and that the World Health Organization has recognized acupuncture as a treatment for neurologic and orthopedic disorders.[6]

In *Acupuncture in Medical Practice,* Louise Wensel, M.D., reported that of the more than 10,000 patients treated at the Washington Acupuncture Center for various forms of arthritis, more than 80 percent had significant improvement. Patients might need five or six acupuncture treatments before experiencing relief, but most experienced significant reduction in pain, swelling, and stiffness by the time they had had six to ten treatments; and some remained symptom-free for more than five years thereafter. People with severe rheumatoid arthritis in some cases remained nearly symptom-free with maintenance treatments weekly or less often. The main treatment point for arthritis, noted Dr. Wensel, is near the hip joint, where branches of nerves converge.[7]

Dr. William Cargile, chairman of research of the American Association of Acupuncture, also cites cases in which acupuncture has helped relieve rheumatoid arthritis. He explains RA as resulting from an inability of white blood cells to recognize the joint surface as "self" instead of "not self." Acupuncture reduces the aggressiveness of the body against its own tissues and aids recognition of the joint surface as part of itself. Acupuncture is aimed not just at the particular affected joints but at the whole body. Particularly important in RA is the spleen, which produces white blood cells and plays an important role in the lymphatic system.[8]

Several studies have shown that acupuncture also improves pain control and sleep quality for fibromyalgia victims, and that it can offer long-lasting pain relief for many of them.[9]

Acupuncture is even becoming popular with owners of arthritic dogs. Instead of traditional acupuncture needles, tiny gold beads may be permanently implanted in the animals. The beads continuously stimulate the acupuncture points, eliminating the need for repeated needlings. While the effectiveness of this treatment hasn't been proven in controlled trials, the fact that dog owners are willing to pay $45 to $350 for the procedure suggests it is having objectively assessable effects on the animals' arthritic joints.[10]

RESOURCES

The American Academy of Medical Acupuncture offers a free physician referral service. The phone number is

1-800-521-2262; the website is www.medicalacupuncture.org. The National Acupuncture and Oriental Medicine Alliance can provide referrals to licensed nonphysician practitioners. The phone number is 253-851-6896. The American Association for Oriental Medicine provides background information and referrals. Its number is 610-266-1433. Another helpful website is www.acupuncture.com.

ACUPRESSURE

Acupressure is based on the same principles as acupuncture but has the advantage that it can be pursued at home without a practitioner. Acupressure involves the same meridians and points on the skin, but instead of using needles, the points are held or pressed gently but firmly with the fingers. Both techniques promote healing through the release of tension and by increasing blood circulation, and both have been found helpful for relieving rheumatic and arthritic aches and pains. For directions for doing acupressure at home, see M. Gach, *Arthritis Relief at Your Fingertips.*[11]

TWENTY-FOUR

Neural Therapy and the Dental Connection

Oh the nerves, the nerves; the mysteries of this machine called
man! Oh the little that unhinges it: poor creatures that we are!

—CHARLES DICKENS,
"The Chimes" (1844)

Neural therapy is a regulation therapy that is less well known than acupuncture, but Dietrich Klinghardt, M.D., maintains it is the most physiologically based of the available options. Regulation therapies correct the functioning of the autonomic nervous system and reestablish the flow of blood to areas that are receiving too little of it. Neural therapy involves injections directly into the autonomic ganglia.

The autonomic nervous system, he explains, is that branch that determines where blood goes and when. Disturbed regulation results when the autonomic nervous system fails to deliver sufficient blood to specific areas over a long period of time. There are only ten pounds of blood in the body. The blood cannot flow everywhere at once. When we're eating, it is concentrated in the mouth and stomach. When we're digesting, it is concentrated in the liver. When we're running, it goes to the muscles. All of these functions cannot be carried on efficiently at the same time.

Dr. Klinghardt offers a common auto accident scenario as an example. Six hours after the accident, the victims aren't feeling too bad; but they go downhill after that. A year later, they're worse off than six hours after the impact. The autonomic nervous system responded to the crisis by contracting the blood supply to the traumatized area, but it's a "stuck" regulation; it never got opened up again. The goal of regulation therapies is to find out where the blood flow is stuck and reopen it. Neural therapy involves injections directly into the involved autonomic ganglia and scars that block blood flow to the area.[1]

Neural therapy was first developed in the 1920s by German dentists, who discovered that injection of a local anesthetic (procaine or lidocaine) at the base of a suspect tooth could make symptoms and pains in distant parts of the body go away. Later researchers found that the injection of local anesthetics to carefully selected points on the body can often cure or ameliorate a variety of conditions, usually of the chronic type. The anesthetic apparently "unsticks" the autonomic nervous system at those points, stimulating blood flow to the area. The result is to flush toxins, at least for a time. Repeated injections are usually effective for progressively longer periods, until in many cases the effect becomes permanent.

Dr. Klinghardt cautions that cure should not be expected in one treatment. Regulation is opened up one step at a time. After each treatment, the body responds by indicating where the next treatment should be. If these steps are followed carefully, however, he says healing can be exponential.

Neural therapy has been extensively researched and is the subject of many publications, mainly by physicians in Europe and South America.[2]

EYE-OPENING PERSONAL EXPERIENCE

I received neural therapy after a dentist pointed out areas of dental infection that I could see for myself on a panoramic X ray of my teeth. There were four of them, one where each of my wisdom teeth had been removed. The shadowed area, called a cavitation, was particularly obvious over the spot where my upper right wisdom tooth had been. Neural therapy was done three times on that area, involving injections of about ten suspect spots with a dental anesthetic.

Following the first treatment, my hip pain was noticeably relieved; but the effect lasted only three days. After the second series of injections, the effect lasted three weeks. Effects of the third injection lasted longer yet, but it was still not a cure.

At that time I was traveling. When I returned to my regular dentist, he determined that the root in my back upper right molar was dead and that its root canal was seriously infected. He performed the procedure commonly called a "root canal" on this tooth, using a nontoxic filling material and the latest in laser sterilization to kill the infection. Remarkably, this procedure was followed by a reduction in my hip pain that has, to date, been permanent.

How could arthritis in the hip be connected to the teeth? Extensive research has actually been done on that question.

ARTHRITIS AND DENTAL INFECTION

The link between arthritis and dental problems was discovered in the 1920s by an American dentist, Weston Price, D.D.S., M.S., F.A.C.D., president and first director of the American Dental Association Research Institute. The case that prompted his research involved a woman patient who had arthritis so severe she was confined to a wheelchair. Medical science could find no cause or cure for her condition. Dr. Price extracted a tooth with a root canal from her mouth, then planted the tooth under the skin of a rabbit. Within two days, the rabbit had developed the same debilitating arthritis as the patient. The woman, meanwhile, began to improve. She eventually recovered from her arthritis and was able to walk.

Dr. Price was so impressed with this case that he continued a further twenty-five years of research in the field, involving hundreds of patients and thousands of rabbits. Being nothing if not thorough, he used the same tooth or shavings from it in a minimum of thirty rabbits (an affront to the species for which he apologized profusely). He found that the diseases of his patients could consistently be duplicated in the test animals, not only by implanting in them root-filled teeth but simply by injecting them with a sterilized powder made from the teeth. Evidently, this powder contained the disease-producing toxins created by the tooth's bacteria. When Dr. Price implanted healthy teeth or sterilized coins in the rabbits, by contrast, nothing detrimental happened to the animals.

Diseases that were linked in this way to infected root canals included not only arthritis but heart and circulatory problems (heart blocks, angina, arteriosclerosis, anemia, myocarditis, endocartitis, high and low blood pressure, etc.); kidney, liver, and gallbladder problems; back, neck, and shoulder pains; neuritis; neuralgia; appendicitis; pneumonia; rheumatism; shingles; eye, ear, and skin conditions; stomach ulcers; ovarian cysts; and intestinal disturbances. Dr. Price observed that angina pectoris, phlebitis, hypertension, heart block, anemia, and inflammation of the heart muscle were often side effects of root canal therapy in humans. Remarkably, these symptoms resolved when the offending teeth were removed.[3]

Dr. Price's work was revived in the 1990s by Hal Huggins, D.D.S., a dentist in Colorado Springs, Colorado. After reading Dr. Price's research, Dr. Huggins added the removal of root-filled teeth to his protocol. He found an initial dramatic increase in patient response; but later, some patients would backslide. Apparently, the "focal" infections in the teeth had not all been removed. But if not, where were they hiding?

Dr. Huggins suspected that they were buried in the periodontal ligament—the "hammock" in which the tooth sits. This ligament is routinely left behind after an extraction. If it isn't removed with the tooth, the cells filling in the hole with new bone will come up against it. These cells are programmed to make bone only next to bone. When they come up against the soft tissue of the ligament, they stop rebuilding. A hole is left over which the skin re-grows. This hidden cavern then becomes a haven for bacteria and other mutant organisms.

Dr. Huggins postulated that most jaws never completely fill in with bone, even after years-old extractions. When he explored these old sites, he confirmed that they usually contained a hole or cavitation under the skin where the tooth had been pulled. After the drill had broken through the skin and bone a couple of millimeters, he could feel it drop down into the invisible hole underneath. He estimated that such cavitations were left after extractions in 95 percent of cases, whether or not the holes showed up on X ray.

To counter this problem, he began drilling old extraction sites as a matter of routine, including those done on wisdom teeth and for orthodontia. He routed out the ligament and about one millimeter of surrounding jawbone, and supplemented the patient with extra calcium. The rebuilding process could take up to six months, but the site eventually filled in with new bone, eliminating further bacterial infiltration. This modification, says Dr. Huggins, significantly improved his success rate with multiple sclerosis.

Other researchers have linked infected root canals and other dental infections to arthritic pains. Duke University researchers have found similarities in the pathology of periodontal (gum) disease and rheumatoid arthritis. Both diseases have been linked to deadly toxins produced by microorganisms locked into root canals and other dental breeding grounds for germs.[4] Infection is a well-known cause of joint pain, and extracted teeth are now considered a major cause of hidden infection. If all of the infection in the tooth socket is not removed along with the tooth, the site can be a hideaway for bacteria that can then impact the rest of the body.

Infected dental roots can lead to a condition called neuralgia-inducing cavitational osteonecrosis (NICO). The patient winds up harboring a little festering bone that never gets well and that can produce chronic, disabling pain in the jaw.[5] Even when the patient experiences no pain or tenderness in the mouth, these "focal" infections can be responsible for "referred" pain in distant parts of the body. The connection is established when this pain, which no amount of local treatment has eliminated, resolves only after the dental infection has been cleared. A chronic painful hip joint, for example, may resolve only after a back molar socket has been cleaned out; or recurrent blinding headaches may go away only after an infected upper bicuspid tooth has been cleaned out.[6]

TO PULL OR NOT TO PULL:
RISKS AND ALTERNATIVES TO
TOOTH- AND BONE-DESTROYING THERAPIES

The problem with extracting teeth and routing out bone is that they are drastic procedures that come with other hazards. They can unstabilize the bite, weaken the jaw, disturb the body's energetic patterns, and result in the need for partials and bridges. Symptoms may also result from overly aggressive manipulation of the jaw during the oral surgical extraction procedure.

Fortunately, new materials and techniques have been developed that can circumvent these problems. Richard Hansen, D.M.D., of Fullerton, California, maintains that laser disinfection can now take care of infection problems without invasive tooth-pulling or bone-drilling. For root canals, the old filling material is simply removed, then the root canal is cleaned and sterilized with a laser and refilled with a biocompatible material. Called Biocalex, this material calcifies the root so that infection can no longer invade it. For cavitations, the threat of infection is similarly taken care of by disinfecting the area with a laser.

To prompt the body to regenerate the area naturally, says Dr. Hansen, what is needed is merely a supply of blood. He suggests that the reason cavitations and root canals are dangerous is just because of this lack of blood. Even a sterile Biocalex root canal can abscess if it is surrounded by an area walled off by calcification where the bone cannot regrow. Like a gangrenous limb, the festering blood-starved area has traditionally been treated by surgical amputation; but the more natural, less invasive approach is simply to allow blood to return to the area. This can be done by making a tiny hole in any layer of calcification that has built up around the infected area. Dr. Hansen has documented cases in which this modest treatment alone has caused the surrounding bone to regrow. He suggests that the beneficial effects seen from more drastic root canal and cavitational surgeries may have been the result simply of the bleeding caused by these procedures in the gangrene-like walled-off areas.

The root canal procedure that relieved my hip pain was done by Dr. Hansen with Biocalex and laser sterilization. For a fuller discussion of these dental issues and those in the next chapter, see Richard Hansen, D.M.D., and Ellen Brown, *The Key to Ultimate Health*.[7] For more information about neural therapy, contact the American Academy of Neural Therapy, 1468 South Saint Francis Drive, Santa Fe, New Mexico 87501, telephone (505) 988-3086.

TWENTY-FIVE

Arthritis and Dental Metals

> *There was never yet philosopher*
> *That could endure the toothache patiently.*
>
> —SHAKESPEARE,
> *Much Ado About Nothing*

Not only dental infection but dental metals have been linked to arthritis. A series of French studies showed that arthritis and other autoimmune diseases can be triggered by heavy metal accumulations from mercury amalgam dental fillings.[1] A number of other studies have also linked joint pains to mercury toxicity. Many researchers have reported relief from patients' arthritic symptoms after dental overhauls in which metal fillings and infected root canals were removed or redone.[2]

The toxicity of mercury has long been known. In the nineteenth century, Lewis Carroll alluded to it when he named one of his characters the Mad Hatter. Felt hat workers exposed to mercuric nitrate were observed to exhibit emotional symptoms including sudden anger, depression, loss of memory, timidity, insomnia, irritability, hallucinations, delusions, and mania, a condition referred to as the mad hatter syndrome.[3]

Cats fed fish containing methyl mercury show Alzheimer's-like brain lesions, and humans who eat mercury-laden fish exhibit neurological symptoms including memory loss, tremors, irritability, insomnia, numbness, and visual disturbances.[4] Mercury disrupts most biological systems as a result of its affinity for sulfhydryl (SH) groups, which are essential constituents of most enzymes and hormones. Nearly all proteins contain SH groups that are metal reactive; consequently mercury can react with many different proteins. Mercury interferes with protein functioning by oxidizing the amino acid cysteine, which is one of the basic SH donors. Even very low mercury concentrations have been shown to affect specific proteins found in enzymes, hormones, and the immune system. Toxicity has been demonstrated when less than one percent of the SH groups in the blood are attached to mercury. Laboratory and clinical evidence also suggests that mercury causes the development of free oxygen radicals that damage the tissues.[5]

Despite its known toxicity, mercury has been used for over a century in silver/mercury amalgam dental fillings. The presumption was that when mercury was combined with other metals and allowed to harden in the teeth, it became a stable compound that would not leak into the body. But clinical studies were never done, since FDA testing for chronic toxicity was made unnecessary by a grandfather clause allowing substances on the market that had been in use for many years.

In 1990, however, the safety of mercury amalgam was brought into question by two new animal studies reported in the *Chicago Tribune*. In one study, conducted by Drs. Lorscheider and Vimy of the University of Calgary in Alberta, twelve radioactive mercury amalgam fillings (a typical number for a human adult) were placed in the mouths of each of six sheep. A control group received fillings made of an inert material. Within thirty days, the sheep that got the amalgam had lost half their kidney function. The study showed that mercury in amalgam fillings is not locked in the teeth but spreads through the body to the organs.[6]

To the objection that sheep, unlike humans, are constantly chewing, Dr. Lorscheider responded that the sheep were fed only twice a day and chewed no more than gum-chewing humans; and that similar data have been reported for monkeys, which do chew like humans. Both sheep and monkeys with amalgam fillings show poisoning of the internal organs and the brain.[7]

The second study involved monkeys given amalgam fillings. The researchers found that normal bacteria in the guts of these monkeys were replaced by bacteria that were able to assimilate the metal. The new bacteria recycled mercury in the body rather than letting the monkey excrete it. According to researcher Anne Summers, "It proves that mercury is 'bioavailable'—something that dentists have been denying for years." She added, "This may . . . explain why not all mercury entering the body is excreted and high levels are found in certain organs."[8]

These studies were dramatic, and they made headlines. But earlier research had already shown that mercury vapor escapes from amalgam fillings in humans, particularly with chewing, and that this vapor is inhaled and enters the bloodstream. After five years, only about half the mercury used in a filling remains on the chewing surface of the tooth; and after twenty years, none of it remains.[9] Correlations were also reported between the number or surface area of amalgams and mercury levels in the blood, urine, and brain tissues. Autopsy studies showed that people with amalgam fillings had twice the amount of mercury in their brains as people not having amalgam fillings.[10] Other research has shown that pulling the teeth does not eliminate the mercury accumulated in body tissues.[11]

Evidence that mercury amalgam triggers autoimmune disorders (a category that includes rheumatoid arthritis) prompted Swedish officials to ban its use as of January 1997. Denmark, Germany, and Austria followed suit, banning amalgams and phasing them out. Degussa, Germany's largest producer of amalgam and the world's largest producer of metals for dentistry, completely shut down its amalgam production, following a federal court ruling that dentists who used it faced legal liability.[12]

The U.S. government didn't go that far; but in 1993, the California State legislature passed a law mandating that the Board of Dental Examiners develop a fact sheet describing and comparing the risks and effectiveness of various dental restorative materials.[13] The California State Dental Board responded with a document titled "Dental Materials Fact Sheet," discussing various dental restorative materials including silver amalgam dental fillings, gold, porcelain, and tooth-colored filling materials (cements, plastics, and composite materials). The Fact Sheet conceded that the mercury found in the standard "silver" filling is a known toxin, and that it has now been shown to escape into and be absorbed by the body. The Fact Sheet also stated that composite (plastic) fillings, the most popular alternatives to amalgam, contain elements that have been determined to be cytotoxic and carcinogenic (cell-killing and cancer-producing). The Fact Sheet conceded that *every* restorative material carries risks, and that patients and dentists alike need to be made aware of them.[14]

Besides mercury, another dental metal linked with arthritis and other degenerative diseases is nickel. The most popular of the reinforcing alloys, nickel is commonly used not only in orthodontic wire and braces for children but in a large percentage of the bridges, partials, and crowns made in the United States. Nickel has been known for many years to be toxic to the nervous system, and its continuous release from alloys in the mouth has now been well documented. Like mercury, it seems to affect the autoimmune system, making it particularly hazardous for people with autoimmune diseases like RA.[15]

Why some but not all people exposed to dental metals wind up with health problems may be explained by the "compounding effect." It was demonstrated in a study prompted by the mysterious Gulf War syndrome, in which returning military personnel experienced multiple symptoms including joint pain and muscle cramps after exposure to toxic chemicals when bunkers prepared for chemical warfare were bombed. The study involved chickens exposed to toxic chemicals. Those exposed to only one chemical showed no outward signs of illness or debilitation; but chickens exposed to any two chemicals exhibited varying degrees of weight loss, diarrhea, shortness of breath, decreased activity, stumbling, leg weakness, and tremors. Chickens exposed to three chemicals showed the most severe symptoms, including total paralysis and death in some cases. This was true although the total amount of chemicals to which the chickens were exposed was the same in each group. It was the combination that evidently tipped the scales.[16] This phenomenon may also throw light on the baffling problem of fibromyalgia, in which sufferers seem to have been propelled into a generalized stress response by a compounding of multiple stressors.

WHAT TO DO?

To determine whether your dental metals need to be changed to nontoxic materials, you should consult a dental or medical professional knowledgeable in nontoxic dentistry. If a dental overhaul is done, it should be done over a fairly long period of time, allowing time to recuperate between dental visits. Dental work itself imposes a major stress on the body. Careful protocols also need to be followed. Removal of amalgams without adequate precautions can exacerbate symptoms, since the patient (and the dentist) inhale high levels of mercury vapor fumes during the procedure.

Merely removing mercury amalgam fillings from the teeth, unfortunately, hasn't always made patients better. It does not solve the problem of dental metal toxicity, because mercury leaches from the teeth into the body. Researchers have found that patients may continue to have severe immune dysfunction as a result of mercury compounds retained in the internal organs, intestinal tract, and nervous system for years after all amalgams have been removed.[17]

Eliminating toxic stressors from the teeth and environment is thus only half the battle. Toxic residues also need to be eliminated from the blood and tissues. One option is the niacin flush, discussed in chapters 9 and 10. Another is chelation, discussed next. Intravenous chelation isn't recommended until all dental metals have been removed from the teeth, but some oral chelators are reported to be safe and effective in removing toxic metal buildup from the joints and tissues even before a dental overhaul has been done.[18]

TWENTY-SIX

Eliminating Toxic Metal Buildup with Chelation

Such harmony is in immortal souls;
But whilst this muddy vesture of decay
Doth grossly close it in, we cannot hear it.

—SHAKESPEARE,
The Merchant of Venice

Although doctors perform chelation with drugs, it is also a natural process in the body. It is the means by which metals and minerals necessary for body functions are transported through the body and in and out of cells. Chelators are substances with extra electrons, or negative charges, that combine with the positive charges of a metal and hold it fast in a clawlike grip. (*Chele* means "claw" in Greek.) Temperature, acidity, and other environmental changes affect this grip, causing the release and exchange of metals, allowing them to be picked up, transported, and released as needed. In hemoglobin (the oxygen-carrying protein in red blood), iron is a chelated metal. In plants, chlorophyll is a chelate of magnesium.

EDTA (disodium ethylene diamine tetra-acetic acid) is a chelating substance that has long been used conventionally as a treatment for lead poisoning. Its effectiveness as a treatment for blocked arteries was discovered accidentally in the fifties, when a physician named N. E. Clarke used EDTA to treat tenants in a World War II tenement house in Detroit who had come down with lead poisoning from the paint used on the building.[1] The patients were all elderly, and many had cardiovascular problems. To Dr. Clarke's surprise, when the lead was chelated out of their arteries, their cardiovascular troubles went away.

Intravenous chelation can also reverse arthritis symptoms. Ray Evers, M.D., a pioneer of chelation therapy for heart and arthritic conditions, analyzed the heavy metal levels in his arthritis patients and found elevated levels of lead in nearly all of them. Mercury and other heavy metals were also high. The link was confirmed when intravenous chelation with EDTA successfully relieved the arthritis symptoms of these patients.

Dr. Evers also confirmed Dr. Clarke's findings that diseases of the cardiovascular system can be relieved with chelation. These diseases are all caused by the same basic abnormality, a narrowing or closing off of the blood vessels. Dr. Evers postulated that the closing was caused by heavy metals that had built up in the vessels. Conditions that were helped by chelation included arteriosclerosis (hardening of the arteries of the heart), angina (chest pain), strokes and senility (hardening of the arteries of the brain), pain in the limbs (hardening of the arteries of the limbs), multiple sclerosis, cataracts, heart valve calcification, bursitis, hypertension, scleroderma, emphysema, Parkinson's disease, and muscular dystrophy. Dr. Evers reported that 90 percent of his patients with these conditions experienced improvement and 75 percent experienced virtually complete recovery, just from eliminating the heavy metal buildup in the body. Possible sources of this buildup include smog, drugs, dental work, and environmental pollutants containing lead, cadmium, aluminum, and other metal residues.[2]

ORAL CHELATORS

Although intravenous EDTA chelation is effective, its safety has been questioned. If done before all of the metals are out of the mouth, those metals may simply be pulled from the teeth into body tissues. Chelation also requires a professional to administer it; it is not widely available; and while it is specific for lead, it is not a good chelator of mercury. There are safer, cheaper, and more accessible detox alternatives, including pharmaceutical and natural oral chelators.

PRESCRIPTION ORAL CHELATORS

Several prescription drugs work as oral chelators. Of these, DMSA (Chemet) and DMPS (Dimaval) seem to be the most promising. A 1997 study comparing the effectiveness of seven chelating agents (pharmaceutical and nutritional) in mobilizing mercury from renal tissue ranked their effectiveness as follows, from most to least: DMPS, DMSA, penicillamine, 1,4-dithiothreitol, glutathione, lipoic acid, and EDTA.[3]

D-penicillamine (Cuprimine), the third most effective chelator according to this study, turns out to be one of the "disease-modifying" drugs (DMARDs) often given for severe rheumatoid arthritis. As with the other DMARDs, the benefits of this drug were discovered serendipitously, without an understanding of how it works. It may be that it works just because it is a chelating agent: it pulls heavy metals from the blood. The accumulation of heavy metals and other toxins at the joints is known to cause joint pain; and rheumatoid arthritis patients have been found to have abnormally high levels of copper, lead, and mercury in their bodies.[4] D-penicillamine may work by eliminating this toxic buildup.

Another interesting finding is that D-penicillamine can be

just as effective on RA patients, with significantly fewer side effects, when given only one week out of the month instead of continually.[5] The researchers making this discovery could not say why, but again it may be because the drug's mode of action is as a chelator. Only a small amount may be necessary to chelate heavy metal buildup from the joint. Giving more could do harm, by leaching essential metals from the system.

The effectiveness of D-penicillamine as an oral chelator was demonstrated in a remarkable book called *Turning Lead into Gold: How Heavy Metal Poisoning Can Affect Your Child and How to Prevent It* (Vancouver: New Star Books, 1995), in which Nancy Hallaway, R.N., and Zigurts Strauts, M.D., relate the saga of Mrs. Hallaway's two hyperactive, autistic children. Their conventional doctors had pronounced the condition hereditary and irreversible, but Dr. Strauts ingeniously surmised that the problem was heavy metal poisoning resulting from a house remodeling and nearby freeway fumes. The children's symptoms were reversed simply by giving them D-penicillamine. A number of children in their neighborhood with the same condition were also helped by this prescription drug.

NATURAL NONPRESCRIPTION ORAL CHELATION

Although prescription chelators are said to be safe, the detoxification they induce can still wind up prostrating the patient. This effect comes not from the drugs themselves but from the toxic residues they cause to be dumped into the bloodstream. The more toxic the patient, the greater the "healing crisis" that can be expected from a detox procedure.

A gentler detoxification can be achieved at home without a prescription using natural oral chelation formulas. Oral chelation is also recommended for maintaining circulatory health after IV chelation has done an initial cleanup of the system.

Proponents say that while it takes longer, oral chelation works as well as IV chelation with EDTA and in some respects is actually more effective. EDTA won't chelate out mercury; but natural chelating agents like cilantro, chlorella, and alpha lipoic acid will.

Cilantro, a leafy green herb, is particularly effective. But dried cilantro doesn't work, suggesting the active substance is in the volatile fat-soluble portion of the plant. Best is fresh cilantro. It can be used as a seasoning four or five times a week, or a pesto can be prepared by purchasing fresh organic cilantro and putting it in a blender with a small amount of water, sea salt, and olive oil. Blend until creamy. Take one tablespoon three times per day with meals. A tincture is also available (the dose is ten drops three times a day), but it isn't as cost-effective as using the fresh herb.[6]

Alpha lipoic acid (ALA) is a natural chelator present in spinach, broccoli, and beef muscle. It can also be purchased in concentrated form as a supplement. ALA binds to toxic metals, increasing the liver's detoxification and metabolic enzyme production abilities. It is a very powerful antioxidant that is both water- and fat-soluble, allowing it to travel to and permeate all the cells of the body including the brain.

The freshwater algae chlorella is a natural chelator available as a nutritional supplement in health food stores. The recommended dose is one-half teaspoon of powdered chlorella per day, working up to one and one-half teaspoons according to tolerance. Dissolve the powder by placing it in a container with a lid that has been partially filled with water. Tighten the lid, shake to dissolve, and drink. Tablets or capsules, while less effective, are also available and are more convenient. (Note that chlorella doesn't agree with some people. If you feel nauseous or start burping it up, discontinue it.)[7]

The chlorophyll in plants is also a natural chelator, and so is vitamin C. Oral chelation formulas are available that may combine a selection of other natural chelating agents including activated clays, coenzyme Q10, garlic, L-cysteine, L-glutathione, methionine, selenium, sodium alginate, and zinc gluconate. Oral chelation formulas have been reported to help with the symptoms of arthritis and autoimmune disorders, among other conditions.[8] Results may be noticeable in several weeks; but since oral chelators are all natural nutrients, they are beneficial if taken for longer periods, and food sources can be made a regular part of the diet.

As with prescription chelators, cleansing reactions may be experienced from oral chelation, including irritability, headaches, and overall achiness; but these should be considered good signs. They show that toxins are being dumped into the system for elimination. Decreasing dosage and increasing water intake helps diminish detox symptoms. When doing any type of detox treatment, it is important to drink at least eight glasses of water daily to aid in flushing toxins.

TWENTY-SEVEN

Homeopathy for Chelation and Pain Relief

*Through the like, disease is produced and through the
application of the like it is cured.*

—HIPPOCRATES, fourth century B.C.

Homeopathic remedies are another chelation alternative. Their
chelating properties were demonstrated in a laboratory study in
which rats were given crude doses of arsenic, bismuth, cadmium, mercury chloride, or lead. Those animals pretreated
with homeopathic doses of these substances before and after exposure to the crude substances excreted more of the toxic crude
substances through urine, feces, and sweat than did animals pretreated with a placebo.[1]

Animal studies are particularly compelling because they
eliminate the placebo effect. Critics charge that homeopathic
remedies can act *only* as placebos, because they contain no
detectable active ingredients. In 1988, the FDA removed a
homeopathic diet aid called Appetoff from the market although
research showed that 91.6 percent of people using it for at least
a week lost weight, charging that the product must be fraudu-
lent because no active ingredients could be detected in it.[2]

Homeopaths counter that the effect of their remedies is electromagnetic rather than chemical. Homeopathic medicines are made by preparing a mother tincture from a particular symptom-provoking substance. The tincture is "potentized," or increased in potency, by diluting and succussing (shaking vigorously in a particular way). The succussion transmits the energy pattern of the original substance to the neutral matter in which it was diluted (usually water and alcohol). The more succussion and dilution, the stronger the energetic fields, since the farther apart the molecules are, the stronger the vibrational resonance between them.

The mother tincture has a potency of 1x. To raise the potency from 1x to 2x, one part of the 1x solution is mixed with nine parts of alcohol and succussed. To raise 2x to 3x, one part of the 2x solution is diluted with nine parts of alcohol and succussed. The process is repeated until the desired potency is reached. The "x" indicates dilution by 10. "C" indicates dilution by 100. "M" indicates dilution by 1000. Homeopaths agree that at higher potencies, these remedies are so dilute that they are statistically unlikely to contain any of the original active ingredient.

That fact caused homeopathy to be discredited by Western medical scientists, since there was no recognized means by which it could work. Many drugs, however, are in use for which the mechanism is not known. Aspirin was on the market for nearly a century before its mechanism was understood. The fact is that homeopathy does seem to work. This was shown in a puzzling but dramatic study published in June 1988 in the British publication *Nature,* a journal that is prominent and respected in the scientific community. It involved a special type of white blood cell which, when exposed to a particular antibody, is known to change chemically and structurally in a detectable way. In the experiment, these anticipated chemical and structural changes did occur. Yet the antibody had been diluted to 1 part per 10 to the 120th parts of distilled water—again so dilute that no molecule of the original active ingredient was likely to be left in the portion tested. The results were so foreign to conventional theory that the editors themselves felt compelled to say they didn't believe them—although the study was performed by reputable researchers in six different laboratories at four major universities, in France, Israel, Italy, and Canada—and was repeated *seventy* times.[3]

Since then, a compelling series of carefully controlled studies has shown that homeopathy has merit. In September 1997, the British medical journal *Lancet* reported the results of a meta-analysis (a systematic review of a body of research) of eighty-nine blinded, randomized, placebo-controlled clinical trials of homeopathy. It found that the homeopathic medicines used in those studies had an average effect that was 2.45 times greater than placebos. For comparative purposes, in a meta-analysis of twenty well-controlled studies of popular antidepressant medicines, the drugs were found to be only 1.3 times as effective as placebos.[4]

HISTORY AND TRIBULATIONS OF THE HOMEOPATHIC APPROACH

Homeopathic remedies consist of heavily diluted doses of natural substances (mineral, plant, or animal) that if given to healthy people in larger doses would cause the symptoms the patient is experiencing. The principle is the same as for pharmaceutical vaccination, but vaccines are macromolecules that can induce unwanted side effects. Homeopathic remedies are without side effects because they are so heavily diluted.

While the homeopathic principle of "like cures like" goes back to Hippocrates, the concept was popularized by the German physician Samuel Hahnemann in the 1790s. (Homeopathic historians point out that this was the same decade George Washington died of overzealous bloodletting and mercury poisoning at the hands of conventional doctors treating him for a sore throat.) Hahnemann noticed that people who took quinine developed malaria symptoms. He also noticed that people with malaria who were treated with minute doses of quinine recovered, not only in record time but without side effects. He then did a series of "provings" demonstrating similar effects for a wide range of substances and symptoms. In the great cholera epidemic of the 1830s, Hahnemann's remedies proved notably more effective than conventional treatment, and his fame spread. Homeopathy has been widely accepted and practiced in Europe ever since and is now the leading alternative therapy used there.

In the United States, recognition came more slowly. Homeopathy established medical societies and colleges in a growing number of states by the mid-nineteenth century; and in 1844, the American Institute of Homeopathy was organized as the first national medical society. But opposition mounted when allopathic doctors saw homeopathy as a threat to their own market and counterattacked by forming the American Medical Association (AMA). Its campaign was so effective that the ten thousand homeopaths and twenty homeopathic medical schools existing at the beginning of the twentieth century were reduced to less than six hundred homeopaths and no exclusively homeopathic schools by the second half of that century.[5]

Today, however, homeopathy is rapidly regaining popularity. Sales of homeopathic remedies are increasing by about 20 percent a year. Partly this is a result of new research establishing homeopathy's validity. Homeopathy is also part of a recent medical self-care movement in America, which has as its goal empowering people to heal themselves knowledgeably without reliance on doctors.

HOMEOPATHIC CHELATORS

A new line of combination homeopathic products has been designed specifically for neutralizing heavy metal poisoning, dental work, and environmental toxins. Unlike IV chelation, homeopathic detox remedies may be taken safely and with good effect even before mercury and other metals have been removed from the teeth. Supplemental zinc is also recommended, to help counteract mercury and nickel absorption.[6]

Deseret Biologicals makes a homeopathic remedy called Oratox which is recommended for two or three weeks after dental work. Other Deseret Biologicals homeopathic remedies in the detox line include Enviroclenz and Metox. The company is located in Salt Lake City and supplies remedies by mail (telephone 800-827-9529). Apex in Glendale, California (telephone 818-243-5336), also makes a homeopathic remedy called Mercury Antitox that helps clear mercury from body tissues after its removal from the teeth. Other combination homeopathic detox products are Dental Detox and Amalgam by PHP.

In my own case, these products had a rather remarkable effect on my arthritic hip at a time when it was keeping me awake nights. I took several drops of the three Deseret detox remedies and immediately slept through the night. The remedies gave me cleansing reactions (a headache and upset stomach)—not bad ones, but they were uncomfortable, rather like PMS. However, I found that these reactions could be avoided by using other detox procedures to speed the process. One was the niacin flush, which helped move toxins quickly through the body. The flush from the niacin was at the same time reduced, apparently because the homeopathic remedies helped speed the cleansing process. Clay poultices helped it along more.

HOMEOPATHIC REMEDIES
FOR ARTHRITIC SYMPTOMS

Other homeopathic remedies are recommended specifically for arthritis. Jonathan Wright, M.D., a popular writer in the alternative health care field, recommends these homeopathic remedies for joint pain, depending on symptoms and constitutional type:

Rhus Toxicodendron 6c for pain aggravated on first moving that improves with continued motion. The recommended regimen is one dose three times daily for three weeks.

Ruta Graveolens 6c for pain mainly involving the large joints; for feelings of stiffness and bruising; for pain that is worse at night and when cold. Take one dose three times daily for up to two weeks.

Ledum 6c for pain in the smaller joints (toes, fingers, wrists). Take one dose four times daily for two weeks.

Belladonna 6c for pulsing pain with obvious heat and redness. Take one dose daily for two weeks.

Apis Mellifica 6c for acute conditions with redness and swelling, or for stinging pain. Take one dose three times daily for two weeks.

Bryonia 6c for severe, throbbing pain aggravated by movement; for pain that feels better with pressure or resting. Take one dose three times daily for up to two weeks.

Pulsatilla 6c for pain that moves from one joint to another, and that feels worse when starting to move. Take one dose three times daily for up to two weeks.

A preparation called Arthritis by BHI is a combination homeopathic that can also help alleviate pain and swelling. Trauma by CompliMed is a topical homeopathic combination cream effective in relieving inflammation and pain.

For an acute attack of gout, an excellent homeopathic regimen includes the remedies *Belladonna* 6c, *Colchicum* 6c, and *Nux Vomica* 6c. Take them as follows: three tablets of *Belladonna* 6c, followed thirty to sixty minutes later with three tablets of *Colchicum* 6c, followed thirty minutes later with three tablets of *Nux Vomica* 6c. Acute attacks are generally relieved in about two hours. Repeat this routine two to three times daily for three days.

A homeopathic remedy with general application as a natural pain reliever is *Hypericum* 30c. Users report that it can reduce inflammation as well as aspirin, without the risk of side effects. Take three pills four times daily.

RESEARCH ON HOMEOPATHIC TREATMENT OF ARTHRITIS

Studies demonstrating the effectiveness of homeopathy on arthritis include the following:

In a British study, forty-one patients with rheumatoid arthritis were treated with high doses of aspirin (3.9 grams per day). The results were then compared with fifty-four similar patients treated with homeopathic remedies. Both groups were also compared with one hundred patients receiving a placebo. The patients receiving homeopathic remedies did better than those receiving either aspirin or a placebo, and they experienced no toxic effects.[7]

In a second British study, twenty-three patients with rheumatoid arthritis who were on orthodox anti-inflammatory treatment plus homeopathy were compared with a similar group of twenty-three patients on orthodox treatment plus a placebo. A significant improvement in subjective pain, articular index, stiffness, and grip strength was reported for those patients receiving homeopathic remedies, while no significant change occurred in the patients receiving the placebo.[8]

British studies have also shown that the homeopathic remedy *Rhus Toxicodendron* is effective in reducing the pain of fibromyalgia.[9]

Dana Ullman, M.P.H., in *The Consumer's Guide to Homeopathy,* cites several other studies involving rheumatic disorders, rheumatoid arthritis, and fibromyalgia, in which successful results were reported for homeopathic treatment.[10]

HOME TREATMENT

Homeopathic remedies are available without a prescription; but unless you were brought up in a homeopathic family, you may have trouble knowing which to use without professional help. Your pharmacist is legally authorized to help you select among them, but most pharmacists know little about them. If you are choosing your own remedies, you need to either read up and become well informed, or choose one of the prepared combination products that are more likely to be effective on a range of symptom complexes.

When choosing your own remedies, you should take only 3x to 30x potencies, nothing higher. Don't worry if your symptoms get worse before they get better; that's what they're supposed to do. This effect is the "healing crisis" that shows the remedy is encouraging your body's own housecleaning efforts. Where conventional medicine suppresses symptoms, homeopaths encourage them, on the theory that they represent the body's attempt to flush out toxins. Coughing, sneezing, diarrhea, vomiting, and skin eruptions are all purging techniques of the body. You should stop taking the remedy when symptoms get better, since continuing with it thereafter can cause them to recur.

Homeopathic remedies should not be touched with the hands but rather just dropped from the bottle or dropper under the tongue. (The bottles are specially designed for this.) Touching them with the hands may "antidote" them, or render them ineffective by affecting their energetic qualities. So may severe temperatures, coffee, alcohol, and camphor-containing products, including Vick's VapoRub, tiger balm, white flower oil, Noxzema creams, and BenGay. (If in doubt, read the label.) Worse yet are steroid drugs, which work by an opposing system. Steroids suppress the immune system's efforts to heal the body, while homeopathic remedies encourage it to regain its original vitality.

You may be able to find a practitioner in your area through the National Center for Homeopathy in Alexandria, Virginia, telephone 703-548-7790. Like other holistic practitioners, however, the majority of homeopaths remain unlisted. Your best options are to ask around or call a company that makes homeopathic products for referrals. For further discussion, see Dr. Lynne Walker and Ellen Brown, *Nature's Pharmacy* (Paramus, New Jersey: Prentice Hall, 1998).

TWENTY-EIGHT

Dealing with the Stress Factor: Nonarthritic Thinking

The body is the instrument of the soul. If the piano player is sick, does it help to repair his or her piano? . . . [R]epair at that level cannot cure what caused the breakdown.

—GARY ZUKAV,
The Seat of the Soul[1]

After toxic blockages have been eliminated and nutrients needed for repair have been supplied, a more subtle element still needs to be addressed before the healing energies can flow and health can be maintained. These are the low-grade negative emotions that feed a steady stream of tightening, contracting, cell-destructive adrenaline into the system.

The study of the mind/body connection in disease has become a science, called psychoneuroimmunology. The connection is now well accepted for diseases such as hypertension, digestive ailments, and heart disease. But what about arthritis? If it is indeed caused simply by physical wear and tear on the joints, emotional states should have nothing to do with it. Yet a growing body of research now links arthritis, like many other chronic degenerative diseases, to the negative emotions collectively denominated "stress."

Most of the studies comparing stress levels to arthritis incidence have involved rheumatoid arthritis. Stress causes the pituitary gland to release the hormone prolactin, which triggers swelling in the joints. In an Arizona study of 100 people with rheumatoid arthritis, levels of prolactin were twice as high among people reporting high degrees of interpersonal stress as among those not stressed. Other studies have shown that prolactin migrates to the joints, where it starts a cascade of events that lead to swelling, pain, and tenderness. The hormone released during stress has thus been implicated in the very thing that causes arthritis pain, swollen joints.[2]

Though less well documented, osteoarthritis has also been linked to stress. A 1997 Finnish study followed farmers who were initially healthy. Psychological distress was linked with a 55 percent increase in the risk of suffering from osteoarthritis of the knee ten years later.[3] In a 1998 British study of 4,057 people aged forty to seventy-nine surveyed by mail, disability from knee pain was also strongly associated with psychological stress.[4]

A sense of being stressed by the routine hassles of daily life has been found to be a better predictor of health status in elderly patients with osteoarthritis than major life-change events (death, divorce, bankruptcy). The critical measure was found to be not the *number* of hassles but the *sense* of being hassled. It correlated directly with physical measures of health status, while the major traumatic stressors correlated only indirectly; they just added to the overall sense of being hassled.[5]

Other research suggests it is not stress itself but the inability to cope with it that is immune-suppressive. In a study at Carleton University in Ontario, Canada, experimental tumors were induced in three groups of rats. One group was given a painful electric shock over which it had no control. Another

group got the same amount of electric shock but had the ability to turn it off. The third group got no shock. The animals in
the first group developed tumors and died more rapidly than
those in the second group. Those in the second group, who
could turn the shock off, fared no worse than rats getting no
shock at all.[6]

THE STRESS RESPONSE

The stress response was discovered and mapped by Hans Selye,
M.D., in the 1950s. He showed that animals react to stress by
releasing adrenaline in preparation for "fight or flight." Dr.
Selye called the entire stress response the "General Adaptation
Syndrome." He found that it evolved through three stages: the
alarm reaction, the stage of resistance, and the state of exhaustion. During the alarm reaction, the adrenal cortex depletes its
reserve of hormones. During the resistance phase, it attempts to
rebuild its reserve. But eventually it loses its ability to resist and
enters the stage of exhaustion.[7]

During the initial phase, stress precipitates a frenzied hormone release involving the adrenals, thymus, thyroid, and
pituitary glands, preparing the body for fight or flight. The
liver, stomach, and intestinal wall go into emergency mode and
give up protein for energy. Calcium is drawn from the bones
for the muscles and nerves. Vitamin C, the B complex vitamins,
magnesium, sodium, potassium, and zinc wind up in short
supply. In modern industrial society, environmental chemicals
add to the deficit, depleting free radical scavengers including
vitamins A and E, selenium, cysteine, and methionine. Unless
these key nutrients are replaced by sufficient nutritional
supplementation, the result is inflammation and degenerative
disease.

MORE THAN ONE BRAIN

It seems we actually have two brains that evolved separately, one driven by emotion and the other driven by conscious thought. The emotional brain is the animal brain. It prompts movement using two basic emotions, approach (love) and avoidance (hate/fear/rage). The human brain is directed by logic and reason. The animal brain evolved first and is wired to respond before the thinking brain, but the thinking brain is designed to have the last word. The challenge for humans is to master the negative emotions from the animal brain that "lock up" the healing flow of energy.

The human brain is the cerebral cortex. The animal brain is the hypothalamus below it. The hypothalamus regulates the autonomic (involuntary) nervous system. Involuntary activity includes blood pressure regulation, oxygen consumption, blood sugar changes, the secretion of hormones and digestive juices, and the speed of digestion and peristaltic action. The autonomic system functions through two opposing subsystems, the sympathetic and the parasympathetic. The sympathetic nervous system generally tenses and constricts involuntary muscles and blood vessels and increases glandular activity. The parasympathetic produces expansion and relaxation of muscles and blood vessels. Contraction cools and constricts; expansion warms and releases. Thus we say we are "frozen with terror" or have "cold feet" when the sympathetic system is dominant. We are "warm-hearted," "swollen with pride" or "bursting with enthusiasm" when the parasympathetic is dominant.

The sympathetic is the system that is dominant in times of stress. During an emergency the animal suspends nonessential functions such as digestion and prepares to attack the enemy or run away. Adrenaline is secreted from the interior (or medulla) of the adrenal glands, which sit on top of the kidneys. Adrenaline prepares the animal for fight or flight, causing the liver to release sugar into the blood. Noradrenalin, secreted by the same gland, serves to increase blood pressure during emergencies. At the same time, other hormones are secreted by the adrenal cortex, a separate gland of the adrenals. These hormones, called steroids, number about thirty and include cortisone and cortisol.[8] Adrenaline, cortisol, and other steroids are "uppers" that cause cells to age and degenerate.

Fear and rage both involve the same basic surge of adrenaline, cortisol, and other steroids. Whether the animal or primitive human flees or attacks depends only on the size of the enemy. If he thinks he can prevail, he attacks; otherwise he flees. Modern man sitting at his desk, however, flees or attacks only in his mind. The rush of adrenaline meant to propel his body around merely gnaws at his organs and joints and causes them to degenerate. Humans are the only animals capable of carrying anger, fear, and anxiety around with them for years at a time, generating low but continuous levels of stress chemicals that impair the functioning of the body. Animals and young humans may experience a momentary surge of emotion—anger or fear—that causes the release of adrenaline, but this chemical stimulant gets worked off in immediate action—hitting or crying or running away. The emotion passes with the crisis. Children can be hitting each other angrily one moment and playing together happily the next. But adults have compounded this simple behavior pattern with complicated memory and thought structures that cause emotions to become sublimated and to become part of our habitual response patterns. Suppressed fear becomes worry; suppressed anger becomes irritability. Suppressed emotion evokes the same physical release of stimulant chemicals, but the chemicals never get worked off;

and to keep fear or anger suppressed takes additional energy, which stresses and tightens the system. Psychic rigidity and tension—fear of letting go, inability to express emotion, and other subconscious tensions—cause a corresponding physical tension and endocrine imbalance.

The tension of holding back then manifests in tight, immobile joints. This isn't just poetic imagery but is substantiated by the clinical evidence linking arthritis to stress. Dr. Selye caused arthritis and other degenerative diseases in laboratory animals just by subjecting them to sustained stresses.[9]

DEALING WITH STRESS

Ideally, major stressors would be eliminated by changing jobs or relationships or habitats. But if that isn't feasible, relaxation can still be achieved though in the midst of stress. If we can't change the stresses we have to deal with, we can change the way we deal with them.

Paul Davidson, M.D., the medical expert on fibromyalgia cited in chapter 6, observes that it isn't activity that is harmful. It is tightening up or being anxious and fearful about it. The goal is a state of dynamic rest, of rest in motion. Relaxing doesn't necessarily mean crawling into bed. You can relax just by a change of pace. Dr. Davidson suggests breaking the stress response by switching your focus to something you enjoy—exercising, going to a movie, jogging, dancing. Whatever it takes to get your mind off your stresses is good. If exercising is your means of relaxation, however, he cautions to avoid activity that requires prolonged contraction of the muscles and to warm up first.

Physical tension can also be reduced with heat or cold applications, massage, acupressure, water therapy, etc. What works to break the stress cycle for me is a short period of fasting. A number of counseling techniques are also available for pulling up and releasing repressed negative emotions.

Laughter is another option. Norman Cousins had a form of arthritis called ankylosing spondylitis that is normally a progressively crippling disorder. He reports that he recovered just by using megadoses of vitamin C, exercise, and laughter.[10]

POSITIVE AFFIRMATIONS

Another way the physical effects of stressful emotions can be relieved is to make positive affirmations to counter negative thoughts whenever they come up during the day. John Diamond, M.D., found by a diagnostic technique called applied kinesiology, or muscle testing, that each negative emotion (unhappiness, depression, anger) relates to a specific acupuncture meridian, and that it unbalances the life energy in the organs served by that meridian. The energy flowing through the stomach meridian, for example, is impaired by the emotions of disappointment, disgust, and greed. He also found that an emotion-induced imbalance in the life energy can be corrected, at least in the short term, simply by saying positive affirmations ("Perfect health is mine now"; "Every day in every way, I am getting better and better"). If repeated often enough and made into a lifestyle, this type of positive thinking can actually heal disease.[11] Affirmations should be said out loud and with conviction. The subconscious is a more primitive, childlike consciousness that is persuaded by ritual, sounds, and repetition.

INDUCING THE RELAXATION RESPONSE

Another proven stress reliever is to induce what Harvard Medical School Professor Herbert Benson, M.D., called "the relaxation response." The fight-or-flight response prompts a

contraction, tension, stress, or separating off. The opposite response, attraction/love, causes a drawing toward, identifying
with, expansion, and relaxation. A large body of medical research now establishes not only the degenerative effects of a sustained release of adrenaline but the health-promoting effects of
habitual relaxation.[12] The relaxation response comes from a
different part of the brain than does the stress response. It is a
conscious override mechanism coming from the "human" part
of the brain. To induce the relaxation response, Dr. Benson
stresses the importance of meditation. He cites four requisites
for inducing the response in this way: a quiet environment, an
object to dwell upon (mantra, candle, breathing, etc.), a passive
attitude (in which we are the witnesses of our thoughts, not the
victims of them), and a comfortable position.

There are many techniques for meditating, but they all begin
with complete relaxation. Rammurti Mishra, M.D., in his book
Fundamentals of Yoga, describes a three-step process: fixation,
suggestion, and sensation.[13] First you fix your awareness on a
part of your body (e.g. your legs). Then you suggest that they
are relaxing. Then you feel the sensation you just suggested to
yourself. ("I relax my legs, my legs are relaxing, my legs are totally relaxed.") The last stage, sensation or realization, is important. You must pause from your suggestions and feel that the
suggestion has been accepted and manifested by the subconscious.

Other meditation teachers suggest following the intake and
outlet of the breath. As you breathe out fully and deeply, your
thoughts are let go. As a thought comes in, it is noted but not
dwelled upon. The object is to drop away from thoughts, to
give the "chattering mind" a rest. Locate areas of restriction—
perhaps in the shoulders, perhaps in the abdomen. Then release,
release, release.

After you are totally relaxed, you can start suggesting and

"realizing" positive auto-suggestions: perfect health, peace, love, confidence, dignity, faith. Although the technique sounds like self-hypnotism, Dr. Mishra says "de-hypnotism" is a better word. In Indian theory, peace, love, bliss, and the other absolute virtues are our true natures. We have simply hypnotized ourselves into the limited view that we are less than we are. Meditation is the way to break this hypnotic spell and realize our true potential. Dr. Mishra asserts that eventually we will be able to conquer all pains and diseases simply by the dedicated practice of this ancient technique.

The Christian version of these positive suggestions is found in Philippians 4:8:

> [W]hatsoever things are true, whatsoever things are honest, whatsoever things are just, whatsoever things are pure, whatsoever things are lovely, whatsoever things are of good report; if there be any virtue, and if there be any praise, think on these things.

TWENTY-NINE

Summing Up

*Much of your pain is self-chosen. It is the bitter potion by which
the physician within you heals your sick self.*

—KAHLIL GIBRAN,
The Prophet (1923)

With all this information, what is the best way to proceed?
Arthritic and rheumatic pain is clearly a multifaceted problem.
I've tried most of the remedies mentioned in this book, and my
joint pain is substantially gone; but which specific remedies
worked I cannot say. I've used multiple therapies simultaneously
and am not a controlled experiment. Arguably, the whole combination working together was required—detoxification, nutritional supplements, exercise, regulation therapies.

The first step is to minimize use of the pharmaceutical
crutches that suppress pain but also suppress the body's own efforts at healing. Pain is the body's alarm system—disconnecting
the alarm won't prevent the barn from burning to the
ground—and inflammation represents the body's own efforts at
cure. Before modifying your intake of any prescription drugs,
you should check with your doctor first; but over-the-counter
NSAIDs taken merely to mask pain can be weaned from as
quickly as you can comfortably do it. For short-term relief

while healing, there are natural alternatives to drugs. DMSO cream worked well for me as a transitional remedy for relieving pain and inflammation.

The next step is to clean up the diet. Eliminate junk food, sugar, white flour, and greasy fried foods. Switch to fruits, vegetables, whole grains, and nuts. Eat them raw or with minimal cooking to preserve their enzyme content. Take digestive enzymes with meals and pancreatic enzymes when the stomach is empty. Both can be purchased at your local health food store.

Then look for foods that, while normally considered healthy, might be provoking an allergic response in your particular case. Begin with a three- to ten-day modified fast on water, juices, and broths. Follow this by eating only healthy nonsuspect foods, adding in a new suspect every two days. If joint pain is provoked, eliminate that food for several weeks, then try again. If it still provokes a reaction, eliminate that food from your diet.

Improving your diet can minimize acquired allergies (those you weren't born with), improve your digestion, and burn up toxic metabolic residues in the joints. But you may still be troubled by toxic buildup from "xenobiotics"—residues from drugs, pesticides, fertilizers, and other man-made chemicals that are foreign to biological systems. To eliminate them from the joints requires special detox procedures, including niacin and sweat therapy, homeopathic detox remedies, and chelation. You might also want to see a dentist who specializes in biological (body-friendly) methods and materials to determine whether you need a dental overhaul.

Meanwhile, you can begin rebuilding your cartilage and joints with a range of nutritional supplements, including glucosamine and chondroitin sulfates, MSM, a good-quality vitamin and mineral supplement, and fish oils. Try different approaches to pain management and the correction of skeletal and postural problems, including bodywork and acupuncture. Engage in prudent sunbathing and embark on a regular program of exercise that puts the joints through their full range of motion without overstressing them.

As important as the specific therapies may be your mind-set and approach. Studies have shown that people who firmly believe they will get well tend to recover 25 to 50 percent more rapidly than those resigned to a life of progressively worse health.[1] This may be true not just for psychological but for biochemical reasons, since if you don't believe you can get better you will merely suppress your symptoms with drugs, which will in turn suppress the body's own efforts at cure.

The purpose of this book is to present evidence that with discipline, along with some independent research, creative thinking, and determination, arthritis can be reversed. You don't have to settle for less than vibrant good health. Disease needs to be seen not as a curse of aging but as an opportunity to improve health and well-being. When our joints scream in pain, instead of suppressing the messenger bearing bad news, we should look for the message.

Beyond prayer and positive thinking, psychological therapies for releasing tension and pent-up emotion can help. In my case, I did some Gestalt therapies for releasing emotion. As the tension released from my solar plexus, I felt it releasing in my hip.

I also got into meditation for releasing stress. The Eastern world view sees the challenge of reining in the horses of emotion as a spiritual problem. The basic error is in thinking we are separate, limited beings who must be closed off or protected from others—that we must fight or flee, become tense or stressed. In fact, says the Eastern mystic, there is nothing to be afraid of. We are all one; God is in us and we are in God; and God cannot be sick. Faith in the rightness of things and the love of our fellows allows us to relax, breathe easily, and let our healing energies flow.

It is the ordinary, obvious things we resist doing—eating right, avoiding strain, exercising, losing weight, drinking plenty of water, relaxing, and thinking positively—that will prove to be more effective in the long run than the "quick fix" drugs that don't fix anything but our momentary perception of pain. When we take charge of our own health and clean up our lifestyles, the rewards can be more than mere pain relief. They can help us progress to heightened states of well-being.

My own experience with yoga is a case in point. Even as a child, I was the least limber of all my friends. I went to a yoga class in Nicaragua only because it was taught by my best friend there, and because I feared my hip joint would rust permanently in place if I didn't give it some stretching-type attention. The instructor, Winnie Edgerton, conceded that I was the most inflexible student she had ever had. At first I lasted for only a half hour of the two-hour class, and that moaning and groaning. But after six weeks of endeavor two or three days a week, I was up to an hour a day and actually enjoying it. In the meantime my routine of detox therapies was cleaning the "rust" out of my joints, which suddenly came back to life and started to feel good. After six months, I was completely hooked on this stretching routine.

Yoga is just one of the rejuvenating experiences I would have missed if my rusty hip hadn't propelled me forth. The prods of aging are not to be suppressed but to be heeded. They can point the return to youth.

Introduction

1. H. Shelton, *Fasting Can Save Your Life* (Chicago: Natural Hygiene Press, 1964), page 119.
2. P. Davidson, M.D., *Are You Sure It's Arthritis?* (N.Y.: Macmillan, 1985).

Chapter 1

1. R. Steyer, "For Arthritis Sufferers, Fighting the Pain Becomes a Way of Life: A New Drug from Monsanto's Searle Shows Promise," *St. Louis Post-Dispatch* (February 14, 1999), page A10; J. Mercola, "FDA Panel Votes to Approve New Celebrex Alternative," *Townsend Letter for Doctors & Patients* (July 1999), pages 27–28; The Burton Goldberg Group, *Alternative Medicine: The Definitive Guide* (Puyallup, Wash.: Future Medicine, 1994), page 530.
2. S. Jacob, M.D., et al., *The Miracle of MSM: The Natural Solution for Pain* (N.Y.: G. P. Putnam's Sons, 1999), pages 6, 116.
3. C. Keough et al., *Natural Relief for Arthritis* (Emmaus, Pa.: Rodale, 1983), pages 17–18.
4. J. Lazavou et al., "Incidence of Adverse Drug Reactions in Hospitalized Patients," *JAMA* 279(15):1200–05 (April 15, 1998). See B. Goldberg, "Pharmaceutical Drugs: Your Money and Your Life," *Alternative Medicine* (March 2000), page 8.
5. R. Steyer, *op. cit.;* J. Cashman et al., "Nonsteroidal Anti-inflammatory Drugs in Perisurgical Pain Management," *Practical Therapeutics* 49(1):51–70 (1995).
6. "Toxicity of Nonsteroidal Anti-inflammatory Drugs," *Medical Letter* 25:15–16 (1983).

7. C. Keough, *op. cit.,* pages 176–78.
8. P. Fowler, "Aspirin, Paracetamol and Non-steroid Anti-inflammatory Drugs: A Comparative Review of Side Effects," *Medical Toxicology* 2:338–66 (1987).
9. "Toxicity of Nonsteroidal Anti-inflammatory Drugs," *Medical Letter, op. cit.*
10. M. Langman, "Anti-inflammatory Drug Intake and the Risk of Ulcer Complications," *Medical Toxicology* 1 (Supp. 1):34–38 (1986).
11. "Elderly Users," *Vegetarian Times* (May 1989), page 13.
12. "Aspirin and Its Cousins Ranked by Stomach Risk," *Business Wire* (November 9, 1997).
13. C. Prosser, "Aspirin Substitutes Can Also Carry Risks If Not Used Carefully," *Baton Rouge Sunday Advocate* (February 20, 2000), page 14H.
14. "Aspirin and Its Cousins," *op. cit.*
15. "Arthritis Patients Warned About Drug Mix," *Dallas Morning News* (July 23, 1996), page 7A.
16. See L. Walker, E. Brown, *Nature's Pharmacy* (Paramus, N.J.: Prentice Hall, 1998).
17. J. Foreman, "Arthritis Drugs Kill Pain Without Irritating Stomach," *Minneapolis Star Tribune* (October 11, 1998), page 05E.
18. P. Galewitz, "New Drug to Battle Arthritis Causes Stir," *Washington Times* (February 16, 1999), page B7; "FDA Approves New Arthritis Painkiller but Won't Say It's Easier on Stomachs," *Dallas Morning News* (January 1, 1999), page 9A.
19. J. Mercola, *op. cit.*
20. P. Galewitz, *op. cit.*
21. J. Foreman, *op. cit.*
22. J. Mercola, *op. cit.*
23. S. Rashad et al., "Effect of Non-steroidal Anti-inflammatory Drugs on the Course of Osteoarthritis," *Lancet* (September 2, 1989), pages 519–21; J. DeCava, "Osteoarthritis," *Nutrition News and Views* 1(4):1–8 (July/August 1997).
24. L. Coles et al., "From Experiment to Experience: Side Effects of Nonsteroidal Anti-inflammatory Drugs," *American Journal of Medicine* 74:820–28 (1983).

25. P. Brooks et al., "Effects of NSAID on PG Metabolism," *Journal of Rheumatology* 9:1 (1982).

26. K. Absher, O.D., *New Discovery Proves That Arthritis Can Be Stopped and Joints Repaired in Three Months* (Marina del Rey, Ca.: Health Quest Publications, 1998), page 17.

Chapter 2

1. G. Perry et al., "Spontaneous Recovery of the Hip Joint Space in Degenerative Hip Disease," *Annals of the Rheumatic Diseases* 31:440–48 (1972).

2. C. Keough, *op. cit.,* pages 12–13.

3. H. Valkenburg, "Osteoarthritis in Some Developing Countries," *Journal of Rheumatology* (Supp. 10) 10:20 (1983); L. Solomon, "Rheumatic Disorders in the South African Negro," *South African Medical Journal* 49:1737, 1292 (1975). See J. McDougall, M.D., *McDougall's Medicine* (Piscataway, N.J.: New Century Publishers, 1985), chapter 8.

4. K. Absher, *op. cit.,* page 12.

5. M. Murray, *Arthritis* (Rocklin, Ca.: Prima, 1994), page 3.

6. C. Keough, *op. cit.,* pages 19–21.

7. *Ibid.*

8. P. Airola, *There Is a Cure for Arthritis* (West Nyack, N.Y.: Parker, 1968), pages 29–32.

9. Max Heindel, *The Rosicrucian Cosmo-conception* (Rosicrucian Fellowship, 1997).

10. D. Doyle, "Tissue Calcification and Inflammation in Osteoarthritis," *Journal of Pathology* 136:199–216 (1982); H. Selye, *Calciphylaxis* (Chicago: University of Chicago Press, 1962), pages 406–37. See E. Brown, *With the Grain* (N.Y.: Carroll & Graf, 1990), chapter 15.

11. M. Anderson et al., "Chemical and Pathological Studies on Aortic Atherosclerosis," *A.M.A. Archives of Pathology* 68:380–91 (1959).

12. S. Davidson et al., *Human Nutrition and Dietetics* (N.Y.: Churchill Livingstone, 1979), page 334.

13. D. Barr, "Pathological Calcification," *Physiological Reviews* 12:593–624 (1932), page 611; J. Ennever et al., "Calcification

by Proteolipid from Atherosclerotic Aorta," *Atherosclerosis* 35:209–13 (1980).

14. J. McDougall, *op. cit.*, page 239.

Chapter 3

1. D. Klinghardt, "Neural Therapy" (seminar) (1994–95); see www.neuraltherapy.com.
2. Andrew Weil, M.D., et al., "Roots of Healing: The New Medicine" (audiocassette) (Hay House, 1997).
3. D. Chopra, M.D., *Perfect Health: The Complete Mind/Body Guide* (N.Y.: Harmony Books, 1990), pages 8–9, 171–75.

Chapter 4

1. See L. Walker, E. Brown, *op. cit.*, "Gout;" M. Murray, *op. cit.*, page 27.

Chapter 5

1. A. Gaby, M.D., "The Metaphor of Autoimmune Disease," *Townsend Letter for Doctors & Patients* (August/September 1999), page 146.
2. A. di Fabio, "On the Microbiology of Periodontal Infections," *Townsend Letter for Doctors & Patients* (August/September 1999), page 104.
3. C. Keough, *op. cit.*, pages 184–86; K. Absher, *op. cit.*, pages 17–18.
4. M. Liang, "Living with Arthritis," *Harvard Medical School Health Letter* 14(2):5–8 (1988); E. Choy et al., "How Do Second-line Agents Work?" *British Medical Bulletin* 51(2):472–92 (1995).
5. C. Keough, *op. cit.*, pages 187–88.
6. L. Simon, "Arthritis: New Agents Herald More Effective Symptom Management," *Geriatrics* (June 1, 1999).
7. M. Murray, *op. cit.*, pages 48–50.
8. L. Aesoph, *How to Eat Away Arthritis* (Englewood Cliffs, N.J.: Prentice Hall, 1996), pages 51–56.
9. P. Donohue, "Some Reactive Arthritis Treated with Antibiotics," *St. Louis Post-Dispatch* (September 1, 1996), page 09C.

10. C. Keough, *op. cit.,* pages 22–34; A. di Fabio, *op. cit.*
11. H. Reckeweg, *Homotoxicology: Illness and Healing Through Anti-homotoxic Therapy* (Albuquerque: Menaco, 1984).
12. J. Matchett, "Thoughts Can Kill," *Townsend Letter for Doctors & Patients* (July 1992), pages 626–27.
13. C. Keough, *op. cit.,* pages 30–32.

Chapter 6

1. L. Casura, " '(Don't) Touch Me in the Morning': Fibromyalgia Sufferers Want Natural Relief," *Townsend Letter for Doctors & Patients* (January 2000), page 70.
2. P. Davidson, *op. cit.,* pages 1–14.
3. D. Clauw, "The Pathogenesis of Chronic Pain and Fatigue Syndromes with Special Reference to Fibromyalgia," *Medical Hypotheses* 44(5):369–78 (May 1995); M. Yunus et al., "Primary Fibromyalgia," *American Family Physician* 25:115–21 (1982).
4. P. Davidson, *op. cit.,* page 164.
5. See L. Walker, E. Brown, *op. cit.,* "Fibromyalgia."
6. B. Berman et al., "Is Acupuncture Effective in the Treatment of Fibromyalgia?" *Journal of Family Practice* 48(3):213–18 (1999).
7. T. Hayes, "Local Physician Cuts Carpal Tunnel Surgery Time," *Indianapolis Business Journal* 16:34 (1995).
8. C. Keough, *op. cit.,* pages 58–59.
9. P. Davidson, *op. cit.,* pages 46–62.

Chapter 7

1. S. Saraswati, *Yogic Management of Common Diseases* (Munger, Bihar, India: Bihar School of Yoga), pages 147–55.
2. M. Christy, *Your Own Perfect Medicine* (Scottsdale, Ariz.: Future Med, 1994).

Chapter 8

1. H. Shelton, *op. cit.,* page 123.
2. M. Garten, D.C., *The Health Secrets of a Naturopathic Doctor* (West Nyack, N.Y.: Parker, 1967), page 59.

3. A. Fujita et al., "Effects of a Low Calorie Vegan Diet on Disease Activity and General Conditions in Patients with Rheumatoid Arthritis," *Rinsho Byori* 47(6):554–60 (June 1999) (in Japanese).

4. J. Palmblad et al., "Antirheumatic Effects of Fasting," *Rheumatic Diseases Clinics of North America* 17(2):351–62 (1991). See also L. Skoldstam et al., "Fasting, Intestinal Permeability, and Rheumatoid Arthritis," *Rheumatic Diseases Clinics of North America* 17(2):363–71 (1991), in which otherwise healthy and well-nourished patients with rheumatoid arthritis showed significant clinical improvement from practicing prolonged fasting for seven to ten days, although the improvement was lost when eating was taken up again.

5. J. Kjeldsen-Kragh et al., "Controlled Trial of Fasting and One-year Vegetarian Diet in Rheumatoid Arthritis," *Lancet* 338 (8772):899–902 (October 12, 1991).

6. H. Shelton, *op. cit.;* P. Airola, N.D., *Are You Confused?* (Phoenix, Ariz.: Health Plus, 1971), pages 112–13, 137.

7. H. Shelton, *op. cit.,* pages 117–24.

8. P. Airola, *op. cit.*

9. B. Jensen, D.C., *Tissue Cleansing Through Bowel Management* (Escondido, Ca.: Bernard Jensen, D.C., 1981).

10. P. Serure, *Three Days to Vitality* (N.Y.: HarperCollins, 1997).

11. B. Jensen, *op. cit.,* page 132.

Chapter 9

1. M. Muir, "Current Controversies in the Diagnosis and Treatment of Heavy Metal Toxicity," *Alternative and Complementary Therapies* (June 1997), pages 170–78.

2. W. Kaufman, *Common Forms of Niacinamide Deficiency Disease: Aniacinamidosis* (Bridgeport, Conn.: Yale University Press, 1943); W. Kaufman, *The Common Form of Joint Dysfunction: Its Incidence and Treatment* (Brattleboro, Vt.: E. L. Hildreth, 1949). See also W. Kaufman, "Niacinamide Therapy for Joint Mobility: Therapeutic Reversal of a Common Clinical Manifestation of the 'Normal' Aging Process," *The Connecticut State Medical Journal* 17(17):584 (1953); W. Kaufman, "The Use of Vitamin Therapy

to Reverse Certain Concomitants of Aging," *Journal of the American Geriatrics Society* 3(11):927–36 (1955).

3. C. Keough et al., *op. cit.,* page 131.

4. A. Hoffer, M.D., "Arthritis," *Townsend Letter for Doctors & Patients* (December 1997), page 104. See also A. Hoffer, M.D., *Orthomolecular Medicine for Physicians* (New Canaan, Conn.: Keats Publishing, 1989); W. Kaufman, M.D., *Common Forms of Niacinamide Deficiency Disease, op. cit.;* W. Kaufman, M.D., *The Common Form of Joint Dysfunction, op. cit.*

5. J. Wright, M.D., *Dr. Wright's Book of Nutritional Therapy* (Emmaus, Pa.: Rodale, 1979), pages 236–44.

6. C. Fredericks, *Arthritis: Don't Learn to Live with It* (N.Y.: Grosset and Dunlap, 1981).

7. D. Schnare et al., "Evaluation of a Detoxification Regimen for Fat Stored Xenobiotics," *Medical Hypotheses* 9(3):265–82 (1982). See D. Williams, "Cleaning House," *Alternatives* 4(12):97–100 (July 1992).

8. D. Williams, *ibid.,* citing *Environmental Pollution* 10(3):183–200 (1976); *Canadian Journal of Physiology* 52:1080–94 (1974).

Chapter 10

1. Z. Gard, M.D., et al., "Literature Review & Comparison Studies of the Sauna and Illness," *Townsend Letter for Doctors* (July 1992), pages 650–60. David Root, M.D., presented a paper before the American Academy of Environmental Medicine giving data from the Hubbard Program from 1983 to 1988, showing a 91 percent recovery rate for drug abusers using it.

2. D. Williams, *op. cit.,* citing a study by Dr. Frank Falck.

3. Z. Gard, *op. cit.*

4. Z. Gard et al., "Literature Review & Comparison Studies of Sauna/Hyperthermia in Detoxification," *Townsend Letter for Doctors & Patients* (October 1992), reprinted in August/September 1999 issue, pages 76–86.

5. D. Williams, *op. cit.*

6. R. Knopp et al., "Equivalent Efficacy of a Time-release Form of Niacin (Niaspan) Given Once-a-night Versus Plain Niacin

in the Management of Hyperlipidemia," *Metabolism* 47(9): 1097–1104 (September 1998).

7. R. Kowalski, *The 8-Week Cholesterol Cure* (N.Y.: Harper Paperbacks, 1989), pages 140–71.

8. J. Etchason et al., "Niacin-induced Hepatitis: A Potential Side Effect with Low-dose Time-release Niacin," *Mayo Clinic Proceedings* 66(1):23–8 (January 1991). The researchers warned that in view of the recent increased frequency of prescribing niacin for the treatment of hyperlipidemia, physicians should be aware of the potential for hepatotoxicity with even low-dose and short-term use of time-release niacin.

9. J. Rader, "Hepatic Toxicity of Unmodified and Time-release Preparations of Niacin," *American Journal of Medicine* 92(1):77–81 (1992).

Chapter 11

1. R. Dextreit, *Our Earth Our Cure* (Brooklyn: Swan House, 1974), page 22.

2. K. Hove, "Chemical Methods for Reduction of the Transfer of Radionuclides to Farm Animals in Semi-natural Environments," *Science of the Total Environment* 137:235–48 (1993).

3. G. Bysani et al., "Detoxification of Plasma Containing Lipopolysaccharide by Adsorption," *Critical Care Medicine* 18(1):67–71 (1990).

4. J. Marks et al., "Prevention of Poison Ivy and Poison Oak Allergic Contact Dermatitis by Quaternium-18 Bentonite," *Journal of the American Academy of Dermatology* 33(2 Pt 1):212–6 (1995).

5. G. Danila et al., "The Physicochemical Characterization and Therapeutic Evaluation of Cicatrol," *Revista Medico-Chirurgicala a Societatiide Medici si Naturalisti din Iasi* 96(1–2):57–64 (1992).

6. S. Okonek et al., "Activated Charcoal Is as Effective as Fuller's Earth or Bentonite in Paraquat Poisoning," *Klinische Wochenschrift* 60(4):207–10 (1980).

7. R. Reid, "Cultural and Medical Perspectives on Geophagia," *Medical Anthropology* 13(4):337–51 (1992).

8. A. Just, *Return to Nature!* (Mokelumne Hill, Ca.: Health Research, 1970, reprint of the original 1904 edition), pages 198 and 217.

9. R. Pendergrast, *More Precious Than Gold* (Garberville, Ca.: Borderland Sciences, 1994).

10. The manufacturers maintain that this product may be safely taken as long as desired, even though bentonite has such strong adsorptive powers that it could theoretically make certain nutrients unavailable by adsorbing them from the alimentary canal. The label states: "[I]ndependent experiments purposely designed to find out how much this adsorption would adversely affect the growth and health of experimental animals indicated no ill effects when the intake of bentonite was 25 percent of the total diet, but did adversely affect the health when the intake of bentonite was increased to 50 percent of the total diet. (From *Annals of the N.Y. Academy of Science* Vol. 57 page 678, May 10, 1954.) Since our product is mostly water with only a small portion of bentonite, to reach the state of toxicity would mean projecting the results of this experiment so that a person would have to consume each day a supply designed for 1032 days. In other words, mathematically for the bentonite in our product to reach the toxic level of 50 percent of the diet, it would be necessary to consume a 3-year supply each day over an extended period."

Chapter 12

1. L. Power, "Exploring the Link Between Diet, Arthritis," *Los Angeles Times* (May 6, 1986), page 3.

2. G. Wilhelmi, "Potential Influence of Nutrition with Supplements on Healthy and Arthritic Joints," *Zeitschrift für Rheumatologie* 52(4):191–200 (July–August 1993) (in German).

3. P. Davidson, *op. cit.,* page 85.

4. C. Lucas et al., "Dietary Fat Aggravates Active Rheumatoid Arthritis," *Clinical Research* 29(4):754A (1981).

5. C. Keough, *op. cit.,* pages 98, 113–15.

6. H. McIlwain, M.D., et al., *Stop Osteoarthritis Now!* (N.Y.: Simon & Schuster, 1996), page 177.

7. M. Murray, *Encyclopedia of Nutritional Supplements* (Rocklin, Ca.: Prima, 1996), page 237.

8. D. Sobel et al., *Arthritis: What Works* (N.Y.: St. Martin's, 1989), pages 221–25.

9. Burton Goldberg Group, *Alternative Medicine* (Puyallup, Wash.: Future Medicine, 1993), pages 181–82, 388.
10. C. Fredericks, *op. cit.,* pages 76–85; see also K. Absher, *op. cit.*
11. L. Aesoph, *op. cit.,* pages 6, 45–49.

Chapter 13

1. B. Goldberg, *op. cit.,* page 532.
2. L. Aesoph, *op cit.,* page 137.
3. F. Childers et al., "An Apparent Relation of Nightshades to Arthritis," *Journal of Neurological and Orthopedic Medical Surgery* 12:227–31 (1993); C. Fredericks, *op. cit.,* pages 21–22, 30, 36–37, 42, 46; C. Keough, *op. cit.,* pages 125–28.
4. C. Fredericks, *op. cit.,* page 59.
5. L. Aesoph, *op. cit.,* pages 6, 55.
6. C. Fredericks, *op. cit.;* B. Goldberg, *op. cit.,* page 535.
7. J. Kjeldsen-Kragh et al., *op. cit.*
8. C. Fredericks, *op. cit.,* pages 23–24, 47–61; C. Keough, *op. cit.,* pages 116–25.

Chapter 14

1. J. Theodosakis, M.D., et al., *The Arthritis Cure: The Medical Miracle That Can Halt, Reverse, and May Even Cure Osteoarthritis* (N.Y.: St. Martin's, 1997). See P. Galewitz, "New Drug to Battle Arthritis Causes Stir," *Washington Times* (February 16, 1999), page B7.
2. N. Shute, "Aching for an Arthritis Cure," *U.S. News & World Report* (February 10, 1997), citing Jane Brody article in January 13, 1997, *New York Times.*
3. "Osteo Patients May Soon Get 'Rooster Therapy,'" *Medical Post* 35:34 (1999).
4. A. Manning, "Can Nutrient Combo Really Work Wonders on Arthritis?" *USA Today* (February 11, 1997).
5. "Osteo Patients May Soon Get 'Rooster Therapy,'" *op. cit.*
6. J. Graedon et al., "A Drug to Prevent Arthritis?" *Newsday* (October 13, 1998), page C05.
7. G. Qiu et al., "Efficacy and Safety of Glucosamine Sulfate

Versus Ibuprofen in Patients with Knee Osteoarthritis," *Arzneimittelforschung* May 1998; 48(5):469–74 (1998). See also H. Muller-Fassbender et al., "Glucosamine Sulfate Compared to Ibuprofen in Osteoarthritis of the Knee," *Osteoarthritis Cartilage* 2:61–69 (1994).

8. L. Rovati, "A Large, Randomized, Placebo Controlled, Double-blind Study of Glucosamine Sulfate Vs. Piroxicam," *Osteoarthritis Cartilage 2* (Supp. 1):56 (1994); L. Rovati, "The Practical Clinical Development of a Selective Drug for Osteoarthritis: Glucosamine Sulfate," Madrid, Spain: Ninth Eular Symposium, 1996:4–7.

9. G. Slovut, "Claims Are Outside FDA Endorsement," *Minneapolis Star Tribune* (November 12, 1997), page 03E.

10. J. Reginster et al., "Glucosamine Sulfate Significantly Reduces Progression of Knee Osteoarthritis over 3 Years: A Large, Randomized, Double-blind Placebo-controlled Prospective Trial," American College of Rheumatology, Association of Rheumatology Health Professionals, 1999 Annual Scientific Meeting, Boston, Massachusetts (November 15, 1999).

11. L. Lippiello et al., "Beneficial Effect of Cartilage Disease-modifying Agents Tested in Chondrocyte Cultures and a Rabbit Instability Model of Osteoarthritis," American College of Rheumatology, Association of Rheumatology Health Professionals, 1999 Annual Scientific Meeting, Boston, Massachusetts (November 15, 1999).

12. "Glucosamine," *The Natural Pharmacy,* www.TNP.com (1999–2000).

13. J. Rindone et al., "Randomized, Controlled Trial of Glucosamine for Treating Osteoarthritis of the Knee," *Western Journal of Medicine* 172:91–94 (2000); J. Houpt et al., "Effect of Glucosamine Hydrochloride in the Treatment of Pain of Osteoarthritis of the Knee," *Journal of Rheumatology* 26:2423–30 (1999).

14. "Glucosamine," *The Natural Pharmacy, op. cit.*

15. D. Uebelhart et al., "Effects of Oral Chondroitin Sulfate on the Progression of Knee Osteoarthritis," *Osteoarthritis Cartilage* 6 (Supp. A):39–46 (1998), discussed in A. Gaby, M.D., "Literature Review and Commentary," *Townsend Letter for Doctors & Patients* (April 1999), page 29.

16. L. Lippiello et al., *op. cit.*

17. C. Cochran, "Cetyl Myristoleate—A Unique Natural Compound Valuable in Arthritis Conditions," *Townsend Letter for Doctors & Patients* 169:58–63 (1998).

Chapter 15

1. M. Muir, "DMSO: Many Uses, Much Controversy," www.DMSO.org (August 20, 1997).

2. *Ibid.*

3. *Ibid.*

4. W. Kneer et al., "Dimethylsulfoxide (DMSO) Gel in Treatment of Acute Tendopathies," *Fortschritte der Medizin* 112(10):142–46 (1994) (in German).

5. R. Eberhardt et al., "DMSO in Patients with Active Gonarthrosis," *Fortschritte der Medizin* 113(31):446–50 (1995) (in German).

6. G. Abdullaeva et al., "An Evaluation of the Efficacy of Treating Rheumatoid Arthritis with Preparations for Local Use," *Revmatologiia (Mosk)* (October–December 1989), pages 35–39 (in Russian).

7. I. Murav'ev et al., "The Efficacy of Dimethyl Sulfoxide in Secondary Amyloidosis in Patients with Rheumatic Diseases," *Revmatologiia (Mosk)* (January–March 1990), pages 4–8 (in Russian).

8. I. Murav'ev et al., "Effect of Dimethyl Sulfoxide and Dimethyl Sulfone on a Destructive Process in the Joints of Mice with Spontaneous Arthritis," *Patol Fiziol Eksp Ter* (March–April 1991), pages 37–39 (in Russian).

9. L. Santos et al., "Attentuation of Adjuvant Arthritis in Rats by Treatment with Oxygen Radical Scavengers," *Immunology and Cell Biology* 72(5):406–14 (1994).

10. P. Morassi et al., "Treatment of Amyloidosis with Dimethyl Sulfoxide (DMSO)," *Minerva Medica* 80(1):65–70 (1989) (in Italian).

11. A. Salim, "A New Approach to the Treatment of Nonsteroidal Anti-inflammatory Drugs Induced Gastric Bleeding by Free

Radical Scavengers," *Surgery, Gynecology and Obstetrics* 176(5):484–90 (1993).

12. C. Keough, *op. cit.,* pages 159–62.

13. S. Jacob, M.D., et al., *The Miracle of MSM: The Natural Solution for Pain* (N.Y.: G. P. Putnam's Sons, 1999).

14. H. Cavendish, "Horse Powder Helps Humans: An Animal Nutrient Can Ease Stiff Joints, Discovers Hazel Cavendish," *The Daily Telegraph* (August 7, 1998).

15. S. Ziff et al., *Dental Mercury Detox* (Orlando, Fla.: Bio Probe), pages 14–15.

16. S. Jacob et al., *op. cit.,* pages 40–42.

17. C. Cochran, *op. cit.*

Chapter 16

1. L. Goldstein, "Alleviate Stiff Joints with Hot Sauce," *Prevention* 50:162 (June 1, 1998).

2. "Nonmedical Treatments for Arthritis," *Healthfacts* 19:1 (August 1, 1994).

3. D. Puett, M.D., et al., "Published Trials of Nonmedicinal and Noninvasive Therapies for Hip and Knee Osteoarthritis," *Annals of Internal Medicine* 121(2):133–40 (1994).

4. L. Aesoph, *op. cit.;* M. Murray, *Arthritis, op. cit.,* pages 19–21, 83–92, citing studies.

5. M. Murray, *ibid.*

6. "Herbal Aspirin Relieves Pain," *Catalist* (July/August 1994).

7. *Ibid.;* M. Murray, *Arthritis, op. cit.,* pages 19–21, 75–93; L. Walker, E. Brown, *op. cit.*

Chapter 17

1. E. Howell, M.D., *Food Enzymes for Health and Longevity* (Woodstock Valley, Conn.: Omangod, 1980).

2. Burton Goldberg Group, *op. cit.,* pages 215–23; M. Murray, *Arthritis, op. cit.,* pages 59–66; J. Theodosakis, *Maximizing the Arthritis Cure* (N.Y.: St. Martin's, 1998), pages 206–15.

3. J. Theodosakis, M.D., *ibid.*

4. M. Loes, M.D., "Oral Combination Enzyme Formula for Difficult to Treat Joint Disease," *The Doctor's Prescription for Healthy Living,* vol. 2, no. 5.

5. H. Diamond et al., *Fit for Life* (N.Y.: Warner Books, 1987); J. Mazell et al., *The New Beverly Hills Diet* (Deerfield Beach, Fla.: Health Communications, 1996); S. Somers et al., *Suzanne Somers' Eat Great, Lose Weight* (Crown, 1999).

6. F. Batmanghelidj, M.D., *Your Body's Many Cries for Water* (Falls Church, Va.: Global Health Solutions, 1995); B. Goldberg, *op. cit.,* page 533.

Chapter 18

1. C. Keough, *op. cit.,* pages 155–56.

2. M. Fabella, "Slow Down Osteoarthritis," *Health Facts* (October 1, 1996).

3. J. Lieberman, *Light: Medicine of the Future* (Santa Fe, N.M.: Bear & Company, 1991), pages 70–71; D. Fraser, "The Physiological Economy of Vitamin D," *Lancet* (April 30, 1983), pages 969–72.

4. J. Lieberman, *op. cit.,* page 70.

5. D. Lawson et al., "Relative Contributions of Diet and Sunlight to Vitamin D State in the Elderly," *British Medical Journal* 2:303–5 (1979); M. Poskitt et al., "Diet, Sunlight, and 25-hydroxy Vitamin D in Healthy Children and Adults," *British Medical Journal* 1:221–23 (1979); D. Fraser, *op. cit.;* D. Corless et al., "Response of Plasma-25-hydroxyvitamin D to Ultraviolet Irradiation in Long-stay Geriatric Patients," *Lancet* (September 23, 1978), pages 649–51.

6. J. Ott, "Color and Light: Their Effects on Plants, Animals, and People," *Journal of Biosocial Research* 7, part I (1985).

7. R. Neer et al., "Stimulation by Artificial Lighting of Calcium Absorption in Elderly Human Subjects," *Nature* 229:255 (1971).

8. Z. Kime, M.D., *Sunlight* (Penryn, Ca.: World Health Publications, 1980), pages 229–31.

9. J. Lieberman, *op. cit.,* pages 141–43.

10. S. Berne, *Creating Your Own Personal Vision* (Santa Fe, N.M.: Color Stone, 1994).

11. See V. Beral et al., "Malignant Melanoma and Exposure to Fluorescent Light at Work," *Lancet* 2:290–92 (1982); B. Pasternak et al., *Lancet* 1:704 (1983); D. Rigel et al., *Lancet* 1:704 (1983).

12. Z. Kime, *op. cit.*

13. D. Williams, "Is the Sunscreen Craze Actually Causing More Skin Cancer?" *Alternatives* (April 1993), page 2.

14. See L. Walker, E. Brown, *op. cit.,* "Skin Cancer, Skin Problems."

15. M. Holick, "Photosynthesis of Vitamin D in the Skin: Effect of Environmental and Life-style Variables," *Federation Proceedings* 46:1876–82 (1987).

16. *Ibid.*

17. L. Aesoph, *op. cit.,* page 237.

18. C. Cochran et al., *op. cit.*

Chapter 19

1. G. Wilhelmi, *op. cit.*

2. "Magnesium Boosts Energy, Helps Migraines," *Let's Live Nutrition Insights* (November 1977), page 6.

3. B. Goldberg, *op. cit.,* page 533.

4. K. Absher, *op. cit.,* page 27; C. Keough, *op. cit.,* pages 152–54.

5. S. Lub, "Copper on Skin: Cultural Beliefs, Scientific Data, Esoteric Ideas," *Proceedings of the International Forum on New Science* (Fort Collins, Col., September 13–17, 1995).

6. H. Dollwet et al., "Historic Uses of Copper Compounds in Medicine," *Trace Elements in Medicine,* vol. 2, no. 2.

7. J. Heimlich, *What Your Doctor Won't Tell You* (N.Y.: Harper-Collins, 1990), page 156.

8. Julian Whitaker, M.D., "A Safe, Simple Treatment for Arthritis," *Human Events* (April 7, 1995).

9. "Researchers Present Latest Findings on Pycnogenol," *Nutrition Science News* (July 1997), page 308.

10. A. Tavoni et al., "SAMe in Primary Fibromyalgia," *American Journal of Medicine* 83(5A):107–10 (1987).

11. C. Di Padova, "Clinical Studies: SAMe and Osteoarthritis," *American Journal of Medicine* 83(5A):60–65 (1987).

12. S. Glorioso et al., "SAMe Impact on Hips and Knees," *International Journal of Clinical Pharmacology Research* (Switzerland) 5(1):39–49 (1985).

13. S. Jacobsen et al., "Oral SAMe and Primary Fibromyalgia," *Scandinavian Journal of Rheumatology* (Sweden) 20(4):294–302 (1991).

14. B. Konig, "Two-Year Clinical SAMe Trial on Osteoarthritis," *American Journal of Medicine* 83(5A):89–94 (1987). See also A. Muller-Fassbender et al., "SAMe Vs. Ibuprofen," *American Journal of Medicine* 83(5A):81–83 (1987).

15. *The Natural Pharmacist, op. cit.*

Chapter 20

1. B. Goldberg, *op. cit.,* page 531.

2. C. Keough, *op. cit.,* page 189.

3. C. Tsai et al., "Estrogen and Osteoarthritis," *Biochemical Biophys Res Commun* 183:1287–91 (1992).

4. M. Murray, *op. cit.,* page 20.

5. P. Davidson, *op. cit.,* pages 149–50.

6. P. Doskoch, "Body of Evidence: Research Findings on Six Popular Anti-aging Medications and Treatments," *Psychology Today* (November 21, 1996).

7. S. Whitcroft et al., "Hormone Replacement Therapy: Risks and Benefits," *Clinical Endocrinology* 36:15–20 (1992); N. Laursen, M.D., *PMS: Premenstrual Syndrome and You* (N.Y.: Simon & Schuster, 1983).

8. E. Brown, L. Walker, *Menopause and Estrogen* (Berkeley, Ca.: Frog, 1996).

9. P. Davidson, *op. cit.,* pages 149–50.

10. C. Fredericks, *op. cit.,* pages 136–39.

Chapter 21

1. D. Williams, *Current Nutritional Approaches to Arthritis* (Mountain Home Publishing, 1989), pages 2–3; K. Absher, *op. cit.*

2. C. Keough, *op. cit.*, pages 60–62, citing Lionel Walpin, M.D., clinical director of physical medicine and rehabilitation, Sinai Medical Center, Los Angeles.

3. Inflammation also increased, but the articular cartilage was damaged more by immobilization. The researchers concluded that an optimum balance between exercise and rest is necessary for patients with arthritis, to allow cartilage to be preserved while pain from active inflammation is also controlled. A. Fam et al., "Effect of Joint Motion on Experimental Calcium Pyrophosphate Dihydrate Crystal Induced Arthritis," *Journal of Rheumatology* 17(5):644–55 (1990). See also K. Paukkonen et al., "Chondrocyte Ultrastructure in Exercise and Experimental Osteoarthrosis," *Clinical Orthopaedics* (224):284–8 (1987).

4. R. Salter, "The Biologic Concept of Continuous Passive Motion of Synovial Joints," *Clinical Orthopaedics* (May 1989), pages 12–25.

5. P. Davidson, *op. cit.*, pages 139–41, 149.

6. C. Keough, *op. cit.*, pages 131–36.

7. L. Casura, *op. cit.*

Chapter 22

1. P. Wills, *The Reflexology Manual* (London: Headline Book Publishing, 1995).

2. *Ibid.*

3. C. Keough, *op. cit.*, page 12.

4. B. Goldberg, *op. cit.*, page 536.

Chapter 23

1. K. Ma, "From Acupuncture to Herbs, Some Treatments from the Orient Are Becoming Mainstream," *Newsday* (October 13, 1997), page B13.

2. S. Stolberg, "Folk Cures on Trial: Alternative Care Gains Foothold," *New York Times* (January 31, 2000).

3. A. Weil, "Roots of Healing," *op. cit.*
4. K. Ma, *op. cit.*
5. C. Keough, *op. cit.,* pages 167–68, citing P. Sechzer, M.D., et al., *Bulletin of the New York Academy of Medicine.*
6. "Acupuncture Useful for Treating Osteoarthritis of the Knee," *Geriatrics* 52:98(1) (1997).
7. L. Wensel, M.D., *Acupuncture in Medical Practice* (Weston, 1980).
8. B. Goldberg, *op. cit.,* page 536.
9. B. Berman, *op. cit.*
10. M. Boyd, "Acupuncture May Relieve Arthritis in Dogs," *Minneapolis Star Tribune* (December 21, 1997), page 08E.
11. M. Gach, *Arthritis Relief at Your Fingertips* (N.Y.: Warner Books, 1989).

Chapter 24

1. D. Klinghardt, *op. cit.*
2. F. Shull, M.D., "Neural Therapy," *Townsend Letter for Doctors* (April 1988), page 121.
3. W. Price, D.D.S., *Dental Infections—Oral and Systemic* (vol. 1) and *Dental Infections and the Degenerative Diseases* (vol. 2) (Cleveland, Ohio: Penton, 1923).
4. A. di Fabio, *op. cit.*
5. P. Bennett, N.D., "Toxic Teeth," *Townsend Letter for Doctors & Patients* (August/September 1997), pages 144–48.
6. R. Hansen, D.M.D., E. Brown, *The Key to Ultimate Health* (La Mirada, Ca.: Advanced Health Research, 1998).
7. *Ibid.*

Chapter 25

1. K. Sehnert, M.D., et al., "Is Mercury Toxicity an Autoimmune Disorder?" *Townsend Letter for Doctors & Patients* (October 1995), pages 134–37.
2. R. Siblerud, "Health Effects After Dental Amalgam Removal," *Journal of Orthomolecular Medicine* 5(2):95–106 (1990); J. Pleva, "Mercury Poisoning from Dental Amalgam," *Journal of Orthomolecular Psychiatry* 12(3):184 (1983); H. Quinn, "No

Silver Linings," *The Economist* (February 2, 1991); S. Denton, M.D., "The Mercury Cover-Up," *Townsend Letter for Doctors* (July 1990), pages 488–92; "MS, Arthritis Groups Get Amalgam Calls," *ADA News* (January 7, 1991), page 10; CBS Television Network, *Sixty Minutes* (December 16, 1990); M. Hanson, "Amalgam—Hazards in Your Teeth," *Journal of Orthomolecular Psychiatry* 12(3):94 (1983); W. Price, *op. cit.*; B. Goldberg, *op. cit.*, page 536.

3. R. Siblerud, "A Comparison of Mental Health of Multiple Sclerosis Patients with Silver/mercury Dental Fillings and Those with Fillings Removed," *Psychological Reports* 70: 1139–51 (1992).

4. H. Casdorph et al., *Toxic Metal Syndrome* (Garden City Park, N.Y.: Avery, 1995), pages 140, 162.

5. R. Siblerud, "Health Effects After Dental Amalgam Removal," *op. cit.*

6. M. Lee, "Two Studies Suggest Risk from Silver Fillings," *Chicago Tribune* (August 15, 1990), pages 1–2.

7. H. Casdorph et al., *op. cit.*, page 160.

8. M. Lee, *op. cit.*

9. J. Pleva, "Mercury Poisoning from Dental Amalgam," *Journal of Orthomolecular Psychiatry* 12:184–93 (1983); M. Vimy et al., "Serial Measurements of Intra-oral Air Mercury: Estimation of Daily Dose from Dental Amalgams," *Journal of Dental Research* 64(8):1072–75 (1985); R. Siblerud, "The Relationship Between Mercury from Dental Amalgam and the Cardiovascular System," *Science of the Total Environment* 99:23–35 (1990).

10. M. Vimy et al., "Dental Amalgam Mercury Daily Dose Estimated from Intra-oral Vapor Measurements: A Predictor of Mercury Accumulation in Human Tissues," *Journal of Trace Elements in Medicine and Biology* 3:111–23 (1990).

11. M. Van Benschoten, "Acupoint Energetics of Mercury Toxicity and Amalgam Removal with Case Studies," *American Journal of Acupuncture* 22(3):251–62 (1994); D. Klinghardt, "Neural Therapy," *op. cit.*

12. T. Levy, M.D., "Teeth—The Root of Most Disease?" *Extraordinary Science* (Spring 1994); K. Sehnert et al., *op. cit.*

13. V. Valerian, "Deadly Mercury: How It Became Your Dentist's Darling," *Perceptions* (March/April 1996), pages 32–35.

14. A free copy of the Fact Sheet may be obtained by sending a large stamped self-addressed envelope to EDA, 9974 Scripps Ranch Blvd. #36, San Diego, CA 92131.

15. H. Savolainen, "Biochemical and Clinical Aspects of Nickel Toxicity," *Reviews on Environmental Health* 11(4):167–73 (1996); D. Gawkrodger, "Nickel Dermatitis: How Much Nickel Is Safe?" *Contact Dermatitis* 35(5):267–71 (1996); J. Wataha et al., "Correlation Between Cytotoxicity and the Elements Released by Dental Casing Alloys," *International Journal of Prosthodontics* 8(1):9–14 (1995); M. Grimsdottir et al., "Cytotoxic and Antibacterial Effects of Orthodontic Appliances," *Scandinavian Journal of Dental Research* 101(4):229–31 (1993); Y. Teraki et al., "Inorganic Elements in the Tooth and Bone Tissues of Rats Bearing Nickel Acetate- and Lead-acetate-induced Tumors," *Odontology* 78(2):269–73 (1990); S. Sahmali et al., "Systemic Effects of Nickel-containing Dental Alloys," *Quintessence International* 22(12):961–96 (1991).

16. J. Klotter, "Chemical Contributors to Gulf War Syndrome," *Townsend Letter for Doctors & Patients* (June 1997), page 27; A. Gaby, "Toxic Chemicals: The Effect of Cumulative Exposure," *Townsend Letter for Doctors & Patients* (June 1997), page 31.

17. M. Van Benschoten, "Acupoint Energetics of Mercury Toxicity and Amalgam Removal with Case Studies," *American Journal of Acupuncture* 22(3):251–62 (1994).

18. See R. Hansen, E. Brown, *op. cit.*

Chapter 26

1. See N. Clarke et al., "Treatment of Occlusive Vascular Disease with Disodium Ethylene Diamine Tetra-acetic acid (EDTA)," *American Journal of Medical Science* 239:732 (1960); N. Clarke et al., "Treatment of Angina Pectoris with Disodium Ethylene Diamine Tetra-acetic Acid," *American Journal of Medical Science,* 232:645 (1956); C. Lamar, "Chelation Therapy of Occlusive Arteriosclerosis in Diabetic Patients," *Angiology* 15:379 (1964).

2. R. Evers, M.D., "A Successful Therapy for the Relief of Chronic Degenerative Diseases" (200 Beta St., Belle Chasse, LA 70037; undated).

3. R. Keith et al., "Utilization of Renal Slices to Evaluate the Efficacy of Chelating Agents for Removing Mercury from the Kidney," *Toxicology* 116:67–75 (January 1997). See S. Ziff et al., *Dental Mercury Detox* (Orlando, Fla.: Bio Probe), pages 37–40.

4. *Drug Facts and Comparisons* (St. Louis, Mo.: J. B. Lippincott, May 1989), page 2190.

5. D. Doyle et al., "The Long-term Use of D-penicillamine for Treating Rheumatoid Arthritis: Is Continuous Therapy Necessary?" *British Journal of Rheumatology* 32(7):614–17 (1993). See also M. Hakoda et al., "Intermittent Treatment with D-penicillamine Is Effective in Lower Doses and with Fewer Adverse Effects in Patients with Rheumatoid Arthritis," *Journal of Rheumatology* 21(9):1637–41 (1994).

6. Y. Omura et al., *Acupuncture Electrotherapy Research* 21(2): 133–60 (1996); J. Mercola, "Mercury Detoxification Protocol," www.mercola.com.

7. G. Bushkin et al., "ALA Fights Free Radical Damage," *Nutrition Science News* 2(11):572 (November 1997).

8. M. Pouls, "Oral Chelation and Nutritional Replacement Therapy for Chemical and Heavy Metal Toxicity and Cardiovascular Disease," *Townsend Letter for Doctors & Patients* (July 1999), pages 82–92.

Chapter 27

1. D. Ullman, *The Consumer's Guide to Homeopathy* (N.Y.: Dorling Kindersley, 1995), page 56.

2. M. Beckerich, "Appetoff: Another Diet Fad," *Veterinary and Human Toxicology* 31(6):540–43 (1989).

3. M. Browne, "Controversial Report in *Nature* Supports Homeopathy," *Townsend Letter for Doctors* (August/September 1988), page 378; D. Ullman, "Recent Homeopathic Research Startles Scientists," *ibid.,* page 335.

4. I. Kirsch et al., "Listening to Prozac but Hearing Placebo: A

Meta-analysis of Antidepressant Medication," *Prevention & Treatment* (June 26, 1998) (American Psychological Association, www.journals.apa.org).

5. See H. Coulter, *Divided Legacy: The Conflict Between Homeopathy and the American Medical Association,* vol. 3 (Berkeley, Ca.: North Atlantic Books, 1982); M. Weiner et al., *The Complete Book of Homeopathy* (Garden City Park, N.Y.: Avery Publishing Group, 1989); M. Kaufman, *Homeopathy in America: The Rise and Fall of a Medical Heresy* (Baltimore: Johns Hopkins, 1971); B. Inglis, *Natural Medicine* (Glasgow: William Collins Sons, 1979).

6. See L. Walker, E. Brown, *Nature's Pharmacy, op. cit.,* pages 109–14.

7. R. Gibson et al., "Salicylates and Homeopathy in Rheumatoid Arthritis," *British Journal of Clinical Pharmacology* 6(5):391–5 (1978).

8. R. Gibson et al., "Homeopathic Therapy in Rheumatoid Arthritis: Evaluation by Double-blind Clinical Therapeutic Trial," *British Journal of Clinical Pharmacology* 9(5):453–59 (1980).

9. P. Fisher et al., "Homeopathic Treatment of Primary Fibro-myalgia," *Homeopathie Française* 79:15–22 (1991) (in French).

10. D. Ullman, *op. cit.,* pages 45, 49–50.

Chapter 28

1. Gary Zukav, *The Seat of the Soul* (N.Y.: Simon & Schuster, 1988), page 188.

2. J. Carpi, "Stress . . . It's Worse Than You Think," *Psychology Today* (January 11, 1996), page 34.

3. P. Manninen et al., "Does Psychological Distress Predict Disability?" *International Journal of Epidemiology* 26(5):1063–70 (1997).

4. S. O'Reilly et al., "Knee Pain and Disability in the Nottingham Community: Association with Poor Health Status and Psychological Distress," *British Journal of Rheumatology* 37(8):870–3 (1998).

5. M. Weinberger et al., "In Support of Hassles as a Measure of Stress in Predicting Health Outcomes," *Journal of Behavioral Medicine* 10(1):19–31 (1987).

6. L. Skar et al., "Stress and Coping Factors Influence Tumor Growth," *Science* 205:513–15 (1979).

7. H. Lewis et al., *Psychosomatics* (N.Y.: Pinnacle Books, 1975).

8. *Ibid.*, pages 20–29.

9. J. Matchett, "Thoughts Can Kill," *Townsend Letter for Doctors* (July 1992), pages 626–27.

10. C. Fredericks, *op. cit.,* page 73.

11. J. Diamond, M.D., *Life Energy* (St. Paul, Minn.: Paragon House, 1990).

12. H. Benson, M.D., *The Relaxation Response* (N.Y.: Avon Books, 1975).

13. R. Mishra, M.D., *Fundamentals of Yoga* (N.Y.: Crown Publishers, 1987).

Chapter 29

1. L. Aesoph, *op. cit.,* page 17.